I0161247

# Survival Medical Handbook

Step-by-Step Guide to be Prepared for Any Emergency When There is NO ONE to come to Your Aid

Small Footprint Press

# Table of Contents

# Introduction

*"Care shouldn't start in the emergency room,"*

- James Douglas

We agree with James Douglas when it comes to first aid and preparing for emergencies. A little foresight, the right knowledge, and the determination to help another can often prevent major emergencies and even save a life.

We don't mean to candy-coat the grit needed to do this, nor to downplay your anxiety at the thought of dealing with medical emergencies and other injuries. However, we at Small Footprint Press believe that, of the obstacles preventing you from helping another in distress, the overwhelming panic you might feel is the greatest. We further believe that this panic stems from not knowing the right steps to help a person in distress, along with the fear that you may worsen the situation instead of helping. We understand this as we have been there ourselves; but we have also discovered that familiarity with standard basic first aid empowers you to act for the best outcome with the least anguish to all concerned.

To that end, we've compiled this step-by-step guide outlining common situations requiring first aid, how to prepare to administer first aid, how to identify what steps are needed, and how to preserve life until professional help can reach you. We've included how to prepare for medical emergencies before they occur, and what items you should have on hand for basic first aid and common minor emergencies at home, work, or while traveling.

Our aim is not to overwhelm, but to present you with steps you can take to prepare for medical emergencies, along

1

with techniques that are simple to do and effective in preserving life or reducing visits to hospital emergency rooms.

We don't expect to turn you into a medical professional. Instead, we hope to provide you with the knowledge to assist a person in distress or a life-threatening situation until the paramedics or other first responders arrive.

As times change and natural and civic emergencies grow steadily, you may need to prepare to preserve life and monitor someone who is ill for a longer than expected period as rescue professionals may not always reach you as soon as you hope. For this reason, we've extended our "be prepared and let's prevent it" philosophy toward first aid as well. At the end of the book, you'll find some alternative remedies and treatments that can be easily made or done at home to preserve life and promote recovery.

## About Small Footprint Press

"Prepping to survive a global catastrophe goes hand-in-hand with stopping the destruction of our planet by living sustainably!" Small Footprint Press Company Values.

Small Footprint Press was founded to fulfill the mission of "accelerating the world's transition to living sustainably while enabling you to be prepared should the worst come to pass."

While we aren't Doomers who believe the worst is inevitable sooner rather than later, nor are we of the belief that the end of the world is arriving, we do believe in preparing for the worst while expecting the best each day. For this reason, we work toward promoting and encouraging sustainable, prepared living as an individual. Yes, many would call us Preppers, while an equal number would call us like-minded individuals. Did you know that in 2021 over 45 percent of Americans, both men and women, invested towards prepping for worst-case scenarios? (Laycock & Choi, 2021) We're not just talking about stockpiling food and toilet paper, but also equipment and taking instructional courses.

We hope that this guide will be one that you choose to add to your preparedness, not just for natural disasters or service collapses, but also for those recreational and everyday situations that suddenly turn into emergencies through unforeseen circumstances or environmental factors such as severe storms and isolated locations. In doing so, we thank you for helping to preserve and sustain life while promoting recovery—extending your first aid mindset to not just people in distress, but to the world at large too.

## Disclaimer

This book seeks to educate and present first aid techniques and procedures in an easy-to-understand way using the most up-to-date information. In doing so, we take no responsibility for the outcomes of your performance of the techniques and procedures, whether those outcomes are good or bad. We offer you this knowledge in good faith and understanding that this information will be used only when required and with good intentions.

While we mention certain brand name medications, our intention is not to promote those products, merely to inform you of the brand names we feel most people would be familiar with and which are easily obtainable. Please use the medications of the distressed person if those are known, and your medications of choice to stock your personal first aid kits.

Regarding the natural remedies and medicinal recipes in this book, please read this disclaimer at the chapter beginning, and all warnings and cautions for all remedies.

## How to Use this Book

Use the first and last chapters, You Cannot Be Prepared Enough and Alternative Medicines for Emergencies to prepare yourself mentally, gather your first aid items and first aid kits, as well as your medical emergency kits for members of your family.

Use the second chapter, Good-to-Learn Techniques, to familiarize yourself with the most often used and effective techniques for treating a variety of situations. We recommend reading through this chapter more than once, and to regularly refresh your memory by reading it at the beginning of summer and the middle of winter just before most seasonal injuries usually occur.

Read through the third, fourth, and fifth chapters, Mild Emergencies, Serious Emergencies, and Responding to Emergencies Related to Permanent Conditions. This will raise your awareness of some of the symptoms and ways to respond to a range of emergencies. If you encounter an emergency and have this guide available, you can quickly go through the steps or look at symptoms again. If there's no time to access this guide, that's okay, you'll have your familiarity with the major techniques that could still save a life.

We thank you in advance for the good you're about to send out at times when it is truly needed. Now, let's get you on the path to preserving life!

# Chapter 1
# You Cannot Be Ready Enough

You can't be ready enough, that's true, but you can be prepared to the best of your ability. While our environment and services degrade and disasters become more frequent, we cannot afford complacency or rely on the expectation that medical help will always be on hand or reach us in a timely manner. It falls more and more on us to take up the slack for our own good and that of our fellow beings.

When situations arise where there is no available medical help or rescue, you will need to be prepared to offer first aid. Before we tackle situations and techniques, we will look at how you can be prepared to meet emergencies before they occur.

## When to Call an Emergency Number

When to call an emergency number seems like a silly question, but there are times when you *shouldn't* call an emergency number, or times when even though you've called for help, it may not reach you and the person in distress in time. Imagine, for example, there's been a tornado, your house is in ruins, and your elderly parent has a head injury that is bleeding profusely. Naturally, you need to call emergency services, but in the interminable time it takes them to clear a path to your house and reach you and your parent, it's up to you to offer first aid and keep your parent lucid.

You're not a doctor no matter your level of first aid knowledge (unless, of course, you hold a medical doctor's degree) and no one expects you to perform surgery or long-term treatment. The advice we offer is to help you prepare as much as you can in the event no medical care is immediately available.

Remember, when there's no one else to offer medical help, you should follow the appropriate steps described for each emergency and seek help as fast as possible.

In the event medical assistance is available, but you are unsure what constitutes an urgent medical situation, you will want to check the following list.

## What Constitutes an Emergency Situation

• The person is in a life-threatening condition. For example, they are experiencing severe bleeding that won't stop, severe allergic reaction, a heart attack, severe abdominal pain or continuous vomiting, or it's a case of poisoning or a motor accident.

• The person's condition is deteriorating fast and you believe their condition could become life threatening en route to the hospital.

• Relocating or shifting the person into a new position may cause further injury. For example, they have a neck or spine injury or have been in a severe accident.

• A paramedic's skills and equipment are required to treat or stabilize the person.

• Transportation to the hospital may be delayed because of your location, weather, or traffic conditions.

## The Three Cs of Emergency

To help you remember how to respond to an emergency while keeping yourself and others safe as your assist, we have The Three Cs and The Three Ps of first aid. These Cs and Ps also ensure you do not panic and that you approach the situation as safely as possible.

First do the three Cs. Check, Call, Care.

## Check

Check for dangers in the environment and in the area around the person, for example if a house is on fire, or they are at the edge of a storm torrent. If there is a clear or imminent danger, you may require help in assisting further, or you may need to make a plan to reach the person safely. Being aware of dangers and prudently approaching the emergency prevents further emergencies and ensures more effective and efficient courses of action for you and the responding medics. This also ensures less harm is done to the injured person and to others in the area. The worst thing to do is to rush into a situation without being aware of further danger. Remember you won't be any help to anyone if you are seriously injured while trying to rescue someone who is surrounded by danger. If you find a potential danger that you can easily handle yourself, such as pulling up the handbrake of a vehicle, or switching off the mains in the case of electrocution, don't be afraid to act swiftly if it will make the situation safer for everyone.

Next, if you are close enough, check if the person is breathing. You'll need this information for your call.

## Call

Call for help as soon as possible. Gather information on the distressed person, check their pulse, the scene, and the location so you can accurately convey all this to the response team and other professionals without delay. Don't delay calling in local authorities immediately.

## Care

After gathering information about the scene and state of the person, provide care until help arrives. Use the information in this book to keep the person stable and comfortable until further help arrives. Prepare to use your first aid techniques if needed. You *can* save a life.

## Don't Just Stand There

During an emergency, it is easy to freeze and feel helpless. With a little bit of courage and keeping in mind your priorities, you can overcome that initial panic and slip into your role of first aider.

We understand that some of you may fear that should something go wrong during your care of the distressed person, you may be held accountable by others, including the law or courts. This is where the Good Samaritan Statute comes in. Every state has a form of good Samaritan law to encourage and enable you to offer first aid and other help, if appropriate, during emergency situations. These laws offer legal protection to those who are the first to respond to a medical emergency concerning an ill or injured person. These laws require you to act in good faith and with good intentions, act voluntarily, use common sense, and only offer help you've been trained to give. This legal coverage and situations in which care can be given varies through each state. Check your local statutes concerning these laws.

## The Three Ps of First Aid

As with the Three Cs, we have the Three Ps of first aid that lay out your priorities during your care of the person requiring your assistance. These are tenets that all first aiders and paramedics subscribe to.

## Preserve Life

As the first (or only) person at an emergency to offer first aid, your priority is to preserve life—in other words, keep the person alive. The goal is to prevent the decline of the person's condition. This may require you to perform an action such as CPR, stopping bleeding, or even the Heimlich Maneuver to preserve their life. Later, we will cover the A-B-C approach, also called the Circulation Method, which should be your go-to method for preserving life.

## Prevent Deterioration

Your second priority is to prevent the person's condition from growing worse. This includes preventing any further injury. For instance, if the person is delirious with a fever, you may need to prevent them from moving and harming themselves even more. Other aspects of preventing deterioration may be applying first aid steps, stabilizing the person, or moving the person to a safer location if it is safe to do so. It could also mean staying with the patient to provide reassurance and comfort.

## Promote Recovery

Once you've done all you can to preserve life and prevent deterioration of the person's condition, you will need to promote recovery. This can take many forms, including providing comfort and reassurance, providing temporary pain relief, if possible, and keeping the person lucid and conscious if there is a head injury.

## Prepare in Advance

According to the CDC, between 2009 and 2010, about half of American adults aged 65 and over went into an emergency department. Most of them weren't prepared. (Are you prepared for a medical emergency? 2018). This lack of preparedness can create problems for doctors and first responders who have no idea what conditions they're dealing with or what medications and supplements the patients routinely take.

Preparedness is not just about prepping your family members with details of their medications lists and supplements; it also involves having a plan of action and getting into the frame of mind that prevents you from panicking at the onset.

It is natural to believe that accidents and emergencies happen to other families, or that there will always be someone else to give first aid to anyone in distress that you encounter. Given the fact that accidents and emergencies can occur at any time—day or night—and at any place to any person (even you) it's a good idea to be at least mentally prepared to act. Like in the children's book, *The Eighteenth Emergency*, what will you do if...? While the likelihood of you needing to fight off crocodiles or treat someone who's been bitten by a lion is low, chances are you could need to help someone fight a fever or treat them for a chemical burn. Instead of wondering what to do, take these few preventative steps where possible, and follow up by familiarizing yourself with the basic techniques that are in the next few chapters. Focus on following each step and you'll find that you will be able to deal with more than a few emergencies—any time, any place.

# What to Prepare

• **Allocate the nearest emergency services** as a matter of course. Determine the fastest, safest route to the nearest emergency facility. Inform your family members and family carers of the services they are to use.

• **Create an Emergency Contacts List**. Have this list visible or easily at hand in the event of a crisis. Save the emergency numbers on your phone—as well as on your family members' phones, too—and instruct members when and how to contact each service. Include emergency numbers for: an ambulance service (check if your medical insurance has a specific one you should call), the fire department, the police department, your spouse, close family members and friends, dependable neighbors or nearby friends and family, and work numbers. Consider creating an emergency group on your internet messaging service with nearby friends, family, and neighbors.

• **Stock a medical kit.** You'll need to keep it up to-date and well-stocked, replacing items as you use them. For a list of what your first aid kit should contain, see **The Contents of Your First Aid Kit**.

• **Where to find your doctor.** Know at which facilities your doctor has a practice and prioritize those locations if possible. Let caregivers and others know the name of your family doctor so it is easy to get medical histories.

• **Use medical tags.** Wear a medical tag if you suffer from any chronic conditions or uncommon allergies. Ensure family members have them, too. When assisting a person, look for a medical tag to help you give the correct information to professionals and avoid problems with medication and allergies.

- **Plan ahead.** Invest in a personal emergency response system if you are an older adult or live alone. Some security services may offer this service as an addition to their regular services. Some smartphone apps and messaging systems can also offer this function to alert friends and family. When planning travel, ensure you know where the nearest help can be located and where medical emergencies can be taken. If you are traveling abroad, be aware of regional health risks and, if need be, prepare beforehand. Don't forget to plan how to address medical emergencies arising from a family member's existing condition. Learn what their medical needs might be, ensure they have sufficient medication, particularly if you are traveling, and inform all members of the family of your response plan should an emergency arise.

- **Prepare a medical information list to assist first responders.** Include: your current and past medical conditions and surgeries; major illnesses of your immediate family (parents, siblings, children); any physical disabilities (include vision loss); names, addresses and phone numbers of your health care professionals; all of your current medication and health supplements; any legal documents for emergencies.

- We strongly recommend further study and that you certify yourself for the most used first aid techniques such as CPR.

## Choosing the Proper Preparation for Your Next Actions

Keeping James Douglas' assertion in mind, it's best to take preventive measures against further harm. This simply means keeping the safety and wellbeing of all uppermost in mind. Here are some preparations and precautions you may want to take.

- Dress appropriately for cold weather. It's easy to lose body heat and sustain injuries in cold weather.

- If you are working with chemicals, prepare neutralizing solutions: an alkaline for acids and so forth.

- When traveling in hot weather and climates or water-scarce areas, carry sufficient water supplies for everyone. Ensure everyone is wearing sunblock with a high enough SPF for the time of year.

- Inform yourself about the potential risks of an activity you plan to engage in or a location you're visiting and carry the appropriate gear and supplies for emergencies.

- If you are going to do strenuous activity on vacation, get a medical check up to ensure you won't have any problems.

- If you're traveling abroad or to areas where you need malaria or other travel vaccines, ensure you and your family take these preventatives in good time.

- Be aware of any potential hazards in your area or region—severe weather, civil unrest, road closures, power and water maintenance with outages, etc., and plan accordingly.

- If you're planning on traveling to or in a remote location, ensure you and family members have sufficient chronic medication supplies to last a few extra days, or that you have a valid prescription you can easily refill.

- Monitor elderly family members and younger members for any possible adverse reactions when their medication changes. Do so over a week or more.

- Keep multipurpose salves, creams or ointments in your purse, bag, or car for small emergencies.

- Always ensure your cell phone and charger are at hand or have a power bank fully charged for emergencies.

- Carry a flashlight or mini flashlight in case of power outages or arriving late at night in ill-light areas to prevent falls and injuries.

- Ensure elderly members of the family have non slip shoe soles.

- If you wear glasses or contacts, carry a spare pair with you.

- Wear sunglasses in strong light—summer and winter—to avoid eyestrain and injuries and accidents stemming from glare.

- Carry a spare blanket or warm covers in the car in case of a breakdown or being stranded in cold weather. In summer, have scarves or light jackets in the car.

- Ensure your vehicle is always roadworthy and that the battery is healthy.

- Ensure you and your family get enough rest during busy and stressful periods so your immunity and focus aren't compromised.

- If you are outdoors, ensure you know where the nearest running water can be found.

- Avoid food and drink from unsanitary places or that may be contaminated. Be wary of seafood left too long in the sun.

- Don't allow friends and family to drink alcohol outside in frigid weather or walk home in the cold after consuming alcohol as it could lead very quickly to hypothermia and even death.

● Never leave children, the elderly, and pets in cars when the sun is hot. Temperatures in vehicle interiors rise rapidly and can cause heat stroke or even death.

## Get Your First Aid Kit Ready

It is best to keep two first aid kits—one for home and one for your car. You might want to carry a small emergency supply of pain relievers, band aids, and antacids with you to work. Tailor the kit to your needs and those of your family.

Always use the medications and preparations in your first aid kit with due care, ensuring you are using them correctly, especially if you don't use the items and preparations often. We recommend reading all ingredient labels even on over-the-counter medications as some medications may contain preservatives, sugars, or salts that may not be suitable for diabetics, people with hypertension, and people with allergies.

Assemble your kits or buy them online. If you are assembling your kit yourself, make sure your first aid bag or kit is sturdy and easily carried. It's best to keep your kit in a waterproof container or bag.

## The Contents of Your First Aid Kit

A first aid kit usually contains the following items. Remember to replenish used items, and to stock quantities as per your family's needs, activities, and location. Make it a habit to go through your first aid kit periodically and replace expired contents, ensure the seals on sterile items are secure, and that your personal medications are of the correct strength as prescribed by your doctor.

Keep your first aid kits out of the reach of children and pets. Ensure older children who understand the purpose of the first aid kit know where to find it.

Your main kit should contain:

- adhesive tape
- aloe vera gel
- aluminum finger splint
- antacids
- anti-diarrhea medication
- antibiotic ointment
- antihistamine
- antiseptic solution and towelettes
- auto-injector of epinephrine if prescribed by your doctor
- bandage strips and assorted butterfly bandages
- calamine lotion
- cotton swabs and cotton-tipped swabs
- cough and cold medications
- disposable pairs of non-latex examination gloves
- duct tape
- elastic wrap bandages
- eye-shield or pad
- eyewash solution

- first aid manual
- hand sanitizer
- hydrocortisone cream
- hydrogen peroxide to disinfect
- instant cold packs
- large triangular bandage that can be used as a sling
- laxatives
- nitroglycerin
- non-stick sterile bandages and assorted roller gauze bandages
- oxymetazoline (Afrin)
- permanganate of potash
- personal medications that don't need refrigeration
- pain relievers such as acetaminophen (Tylenol) and ibuprofen (Advil, Motrin, IB)
- petroleum jelly or other lubricant
- plastic bags in assorted sizes
- plastic film
- pocket mask
- rubber tourniquet or 16 French catheter
- safety pins in assorted sizes
- scissors
- sterile saline solution for irrigation and flushing
- super glue
- surgical mask or other breathing barrier

- syringe, medicine cup, or spoon
- thermometer
- turkey baster or other suction device for flushing wounds
- tweezers

You may also keep aspirin in your first aid kit as it can be lifesaving for adults with chest pains. However, you should *never give aspirin to children*, nor use it for anyone who is allergic to it, is on blood-thinning medication, or if their doctor has advised them not to take aspirin and related medication.

We also recommend carrying a pocket mask (a mask with a tube that fits over the mouth of the person you are giving CPR) for your own safety and for easier delivery of rescue breaths.

## Emergency Items

In addition to a first aid kit, you'll need some emergency items that should also be stored in waterproof, airtight containers. We recommend keeping your emergency kit with or close by your first aid kit. We suggest storing the following items.

- Emergency phone numbers including your family doctor and pediatrician, local emergency services, emergency roadside service providers, and the Poison Helpline which, in the USA, is 800-222-1222
- Medical consent forms for each family member
- Medical history forms for each family member

- Small, waterproof flashlight or headlamp with extra batteries or rechargeable
- Waterproof matches or cigarette lighter with fuel
- Safety pins to fasten bandages or slings
- Small notepad and waterproof writing instrument
- Emergency space blanket
- Cell phone with solar charger
- Sunscreen
- Insect repellent
- Water—one gallon a day for each person per a day
- Non-perishable food, including baby food if necessary
- Blanket
- Whistle
- Dust mask
- Wrench or pliers or multipurpose Swiss army knife style tool
- Plastic sheeting and duct tape for improvising shelter
- Soap, toothbrushes, feminine hygiene supplies, and other personal care items
- Moist towelettes, garbage bags, and plastic ties for personal sanitation
- Copy of Insurance cards
- Cash, change, and (if available travelers checks)
- Maps of the area
- Extra sets of car and house keys

- Personal GPS locator if you are traveling alone or hiking in remote regions

Check your kit periodically to ensure batteries are working and safe to use, chargers are working, and items are up to date.

## For Caregivers of an Aging Adult

If you are a caregiver or an aging adult, the Mayo Clinic recommends you know and note the following ten points concerning each senior. (Here are your survival kit essentials. 2019)

- Doctor's names
- Parent's birth date
- List of allergies
- Advance directive
- Major medical problems
- List of medication and nutritional supplements
- A record of the patient's religious beliefs
- Medical insurance information
- Prior surgeries and major medical procedures
- Lifestyle information such as whether they are a teetotaler or smoker

We strongly suggest the elderly be encouraged to prepare and execute a living will, a durable health care power of attorney, and an advance directive. The living will and advance directive record the person's preferences on medical treatment covering various circumstances. The durable health care power of attorney grants the holder authority to make medical decisions on the senior's behalf when they are unable to do so themselves. as well as allows the holder to access important medical records.

## Tips for Unexpected Quarantining

Quarantining helps stop the rapid spread of an infectious disease. You may be asked to quarantine yourself, your family, or even your geographical region by your doctor, local government, or national government. Travelers may also be asked to self-isolate or quarantine to prevent any possibilities of locals being infected by a disease from another region, and vice-versa.

Quarantining can save you and others from severe illness and even death and can sometimes be imposed at very short notice. Quarantine periods may vary from seven days up to two weeks (14 days) or more. During regional quarantines, medical help may take longer to arrive, and some restrictions may apply.

If you find yourself in a sudden quarantine or needing to care for one who is self-isolating, we recommend the following.

## Be Prepared at Home

If you have some notice before a quarantine is imposed:

• Ensure you have enough food and water for everyone, including your pets, for at least 14 days. It is always good to keep a few days' supply of non-perishable food such as UHT milk and canned food for any emergency, as well as ingredients to bake bread and other meal components.

• Ensure you have enough prescribed medication for all family members for two weeks.

- Ensure your first aid kits are well stocked with non-expired items, or ingredients to prepare some first aid preparations yourself.

- Have internet access, a phone, a radio, or a TV to stay updated on official news and instructions regarding a regional quarantine.

- If you are self-isolating or caring for someone in isolation, arrange to call the doctor or medical center regularly.

- Educate yourself on the signs and symptoms of the disease, as well as where and how to get help should you or anyone in your home contract the disease.

- Stock sanitizers, including extra hand sanitizers and hygiene products for everyone present.

- Stock sufficient consumables such as toilet paper, paper handkerchiefs/tissues, antibacterial wipes (or wet wipes). You may also want to include latex gloves and masks for everyone in case of having to leave your home for any reason.

- Ensure you have paracetamol to treat fevers in your first aid kits.

- Arrange with friends and family to have a buddy system in place in case your household goes into quarantine or if you live alone.

- Stock up on some wellness and activity items you and family members can do at home to keep everyone from getting cabin fever.

## Chapter 2
# Good-To-Learn Techniques

One way to eliminate panic during a medical emergency is to learn the techniques that are used in many responses to a variety of eventualities, such as the A-B-C technique, which is used most often and in multiple circumstances. Other techniques also build up the response to effective first aid. We recommend mastering the following most employed techniques as you'll use them most often.

Before doing a diagnostic technique, keep your own safety and health in mind. You will also need to avoid cross-contamination.

If you're feeling faint or need a moment, ask for help, or take a few deep breaths and refocus on your task. Remember you're the best help the distressed person has at that moment.

While care has been taken to set out signs, symptoms, and steps to follow, your discretion and knowledge about the person in distress and other factors should also be taken into account when determining what help, if any, is required from you.

Always be aware of the dignity of the person in distress and do your best to preserve it along with their life.

## Avoid Cross-Contamination and Ensure your Safety

1. Wash your hands thoroughly or use hand sanitizer or rubbing alcohol to cleanse your hands before aiding a person.

2. Don't cough, sneeze, or breathe on a wound. 3. Ensure all cuts and scrapes on your hands are covered with a waterproof dressing.

3. Wear non-latex surgical gloves and a surgical mask if they are available. If not, use plastic bags, or if the person is capable, ask them to dress their own wounds.

4. If you are giving CPR, wear a mask to avoid possible infection or contamination.

5. Don't touch a wound with your bare hands. Don't touch any part of a dressing or swab that will be directly applied to a wound.

6. Dispose of all waste carefully to reduce the risk of contamination to others. Take particular care with needles and other sharp objects. Keep them in a plastic container or similar sealed container and dispose of them with medical waste or as safely as possible.

## How To Remove Objects From a Person's Pockets

Sometimes, you may need to remove a person's phone or other bulky objects from their pockets, or to search for information. To avoid complications and to reassure the person, follow these steps.

1. Ask the person for permission first.

1. If there are other people around, ask for a reliable witness.

2. Once you remove an item or the person's glasses, place it beside them where they can easily see it or find it when they recover.

3. If the person becomes unconscious, ensure all their belongings travel with them to the hospital or medical facilities or that their bundle is handed to the police.

## What Information to Give When Calling Emergency Services

- Your name
- That you are responding as a first aider
- Your telephone number
- Your location
- Type of emergency
- Any details about the person in distress
- Any dangers in the area, for example, fire, smoke, live electric cables

Keep calm and keep your answers brief and to the point. Deliver as much information as you can in the shortest possible time. Listen carefully to the dispatcher and answer clearly as best you can. It's okay if you can't answer the question, but don't waste time waffling your answers.

## Taking Notes for Medical Response

As a first responder, if possible, take notes at the scene. This information will help in the fast diagnosis and treatment of the person when medical professionals arrive or when they get to a hospital.

Take note of:

- The injury or injuries found.
- How the injury occurred.

- Information the person supplies about themselves.

- Timing of events (how long between changes in consciousness, changes in the person's behavior)

- The person's pulse and other vitals

- Any treatment you are giving.

- Medication used, and medication found on the person. Any medications given and time taken.

- The person's next of kin.

- Your phone number.

## Diagnostic Techniques

A-B-C

Once you have determined that there is no imminent environmental danger to you and the person you're assisting, and have checked whether they are responsive— responding to your voice or touch (EFWA Basic First Aid Training, 2021)—it's time to apply the A B-C to preserve life.

A-Airway

- Is the person's airway clear? Is the person breathing?

- If the person is conscious, responding to you, and their airway is clear, assess how best you can assist them with their emergency.

- If the person is unconscious or not responding, check their airway for obstructions by opening their mouth and looking inside. If there are no obstructions, tilt their chin gently back by lifting their chin and check for breathing. If there is an **obstruction**, place the person in the **Recovery**

**Position**, open their mouth and clear the contents, then tilt the head back and check for breathing.

B-Breathing

- Check for breathing by looking for up and down movements of the chest.

- Listen by putting your ear near their mouth or nose.

- Feel for breathing by placing your hand on the lower part of the chest.

- If the person is unconscious and breathing, carefully roll them onto their side while ensuring you keep their head, neck, and spine in alignment.

C-Circulation

- Is the person in distress bleeding profusely? If so, the bleeding must be staunched as soon as possible to prevent the person going into shock. Shock can be life-threatening, so preventing shock is a priority in preserving life.

## Assess Priorities

Before applying any techniques and after checking that it's safe to offer first aid, we need to assess the priorities as the person may have more than one injury and the possibility of shock exists in most medical emergencies.

First

Identify the injuries and/or medical condition of the person. Keep in mind there might be internal injuries, particularly in the case of motor or mechanical accidents.

Second

Treat injuries in order of severity and threat to life. For instance, if a person is not breathing but is bleeding, you'll need to get them breathing first.

Third

Decide what type of care the person in distress needs. Arrange for this care by calling for help or providing comfort and reassurance until professional help arrives.

Check the Person's Response

(Conscious/Unconscious)

• Determine if the person is conscious or unconscious by observing them as you approach. Next, introduce yourself even if they appear to be unconscious and unresponsive. Ask them questions or give them a command. Questions to ask might be: "What happened?" or "Are you all right?" Commands could be something like "Open your eyes!" or "Move your hand if you can hear me."

• If there is no response from the distressed person, gently shake their shoulders. If there's still no response, consider them unconscious. If the person responds by making eye contact or some other gesture, they are conscious.

**Note:** If you have to treat more than one person, the unresponsive or unconscious are to be attended to first. If you suspect or know that the person is a drug addict, take extra care as they may have needles on them.

## Conduct the A-B-C

Run through the A-B-C diagnostic technique, clearing their airway if necessary, and shifting them into the recovery position.

# Run a Secondary Survey

● Find out as much history as you can. Determine what happened and relevant medical history. You can also ask a witness if the distressed person is unconscious or cannot give a clear account. Look for medical tags and other emergency information the person might be carrying.

● Determine the symptoms—any injuries or abnormalities the person describes, or a witness provides.

● Determine the signs—injuries and abnormalities that you can see.

● Use the AMPLE method to question the person or a witness:

● A - Do you have any allergies?

● M - Do you have any medication?

● P - Do you have pre-existing conditions (hypertension, diabetes, asthma, etc.)

● L - When did you last eat, and what did you eat?

● E - Events timeline - What happened?

# Keep in Mind

● Remain calm. There's no need to panic. You're doing the best you can.

● Be aware of the risks to yourself as well as to others.

● Build and maintain trust with the person you're helping.

● Remember your own needs. Ask for help even from the person you're helping, for example clamp their hand on their wound as you prepare a sterile gauze.

## Opening the Airway

• If you see a blockage at the back or high in the throat, use your finger to sweep out the obstruction. If you don't see an object, don't do a finger sweep. Be careful not to push the obstruction deeper into the airway, a hazard with younger children.

• Often, the loss of muscle control causes an airway obstruction when the tongue falls back, blocking the airway. You will want to check if the person's breathing is becoming difficult and noisy, or stopping. Lift the chin and tilt the head back as in the A-B-C to move the tongue away from the airway and allow rescue breaths to be effective.

## Mouth-To-Mouth Respiration or Mouth-To-Nose Respiration for an Adult

1. Ensure the distressed person is lying flat on their back. Clear any blockage from the mouth. Kneel beside the person's head.

2. Tilt the head back.

3. Pinch the nose with one hand. With your other hand, pull their mouth open. Do not press on the neck. For mouth-to-nose respiration, close the person's mouth with your thumb.

4. Breathe in deeply. With your mouth covering the patient's mouth completely, breathe out steadily so all your breath is transferred to the patient's mouth. If you need to fill their lungs, breathe out strong breaths. Look for the patient's chest rising. For mouth-to-nose respiration, put your mouth around the person's nose.

5. Lift your mouth away, allowing the patient to breathe out and for you to take another breath of air.

6. Turn your head to look for the chest falling, feel the air they breathed out on your cheek, and to listen to the sound of the patient breathing out. For mouth-to-nose respiration, you may need to open the patient's mouth to let air out.

7. Take another breath of air. When the chest has fallen, blow into the patient's mouth or nose as you did before. Watch for the person's exhaled breath. Check that their heart is beating.

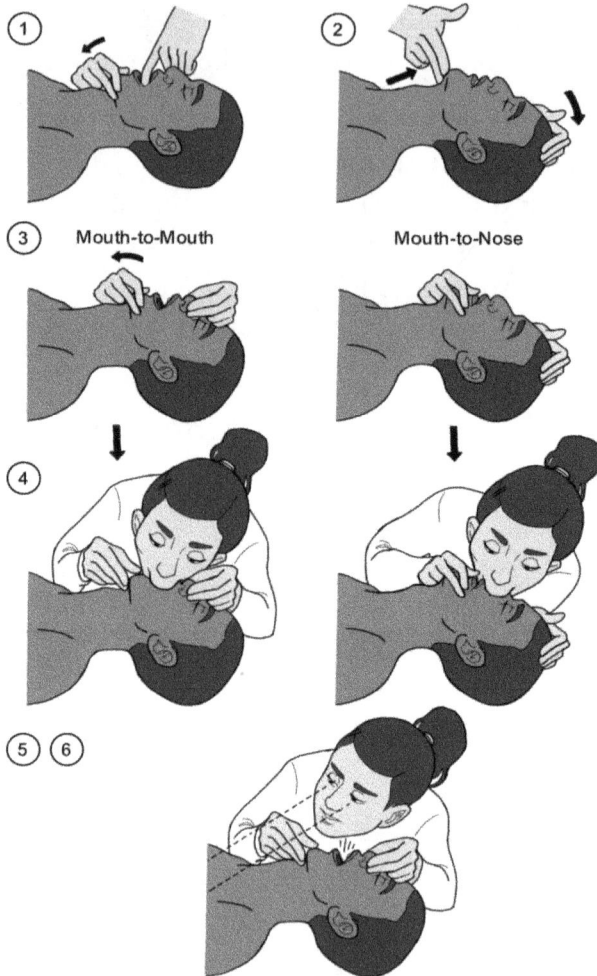

**Mouth-to-Mouth**        **Mouth-to-Nose**

# Putting Someone in the Recovery Position

1. Kneel beside the distressed person. Remove glasses and large items such as cell phones from their pockets. Don't remove smaller items from their pockets.

2. Ensure both of their legs lie straight. Lift the distressed person's arm with care and set it ninety

degrees, or as close as possible, to the body. Take care with the elbow when bending it and set the arm down with the palm facing up. 3. Move their other arm across their chest. Hold the back of their hand against their cheek closest to you. With your other hand, grasp their leg across from you just above the knee and pull it up, ensuring their foot stays flat on the ground. 4. While holding their hand against their cheek, pull on the bent leg just above the knee and roll them toward you and onto their side.

4. Adjust the upper leg (the one you pulled on), so that the hip and knee lie at ninety degrees to each other.

5. Tilt their head back and lift their chin to prevent obstructions to their airway. If necessary, adjust their hand under their cheek to ensure the airway remains open.

6. If the person has to stay in the recovery position for more than thirty minutes, roll them onto their back, and set them in the recovery position on the other side, unless they have injuries on that side.

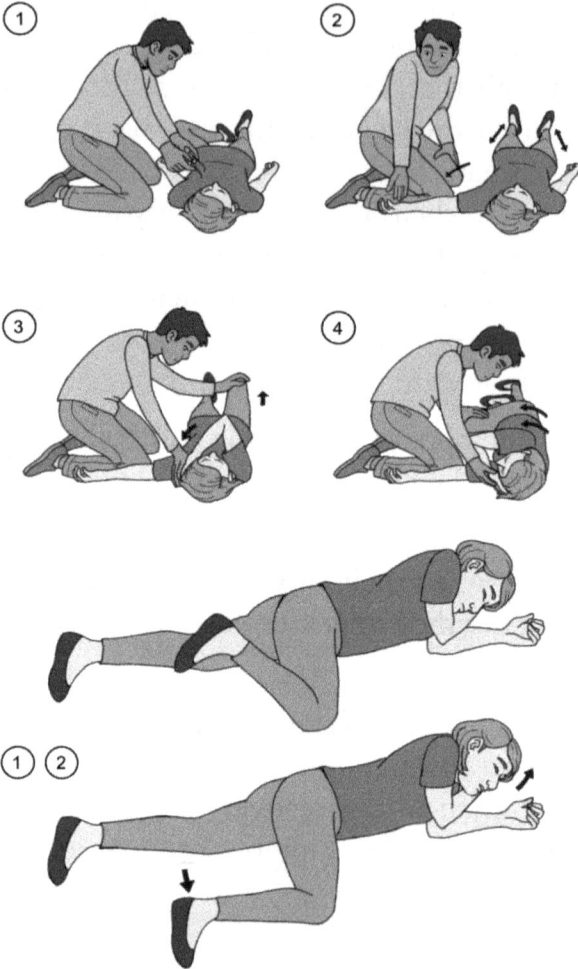

## Cleansing and Sterilization

You'll be using two methods of cleansing and sterilizing the skin during first aid applications.

## Skin Cleansing

Cleanse the skin with a swab saturated in 70 percent alcohol or organic iodine that may be labeled povidone iodine or similar. Swipe the swab across the skin for a few seconds.

## Skin Sterilization

Should you need to cut or puncture the skin, you will have to sterilize the skin so that bacteria on the skin is eliminated, except for those deep in the sweat glands and hair follicles.

However, should the person's life be threatened by a delay in treatment, skin sterilization can be skipped.

There are two methods you could use:

• Use as much 70 percent alcohol as needed to scrub the skin thoroughly for 2 minutes.

• If you have a first aid kit handy, you can apply 2% iodine tincture to a sterile gauze pad and cover the skin till the iodine dries. Use a 4x4 in2 (10x10 cm2) pad. Once you remove the pad, replace it with another gauze swab soaked in 70% alcohol to prevent the iodine from burning the skin.

When sterilizing, be sure to:

• Sterilize a much larger area of skin than at just the site of the treatment.

• When applying the disinfectant, begin where you'll be breaking the skin and work around the area in larger and larger concentric circles.

• Wear sterile gloves when disinfecting the skin.

# Reducing the Risk of Infection During First Aid

- Wash or sanitize your hands using antibacterial products where possible before working on a wound.

- Wear disposable medical gloves from the first aid kit.

- Avoid breathing, coughing, and sneezing over a wound.

- Cleaning the wound depends on the type, severity of the wound, and severity of bleeding. If unsure, clean only around the wound.

- Use a sterile dressing to cover the wound. Avoid touching the surface of the dressing that is applied to the wound.

## Using Bandages During First Aid

Points to remember when bandaging a distressed person include the following:

- Ensure the distressed person is seated or lying down. Move until you are in front of them, on their injured side.

- Ensure the injured body part is supported and in position before you begin bandaging.

- If the person can assist, let them hold the dressing in place as you wind the 'tail' of the bandage once fully around the limb to anchor it in place. If you have no assistance, wrap the 'tail' of the bandage directly around the padding on the wound.

- When winding the bandage around the injury, ensure every turn of the bandage overlaps the one before. An alternative method is to bandage in a "figure eight."

- To prevent circulation problems in hands and feet, ensure that the bandage is not too tight. To check that the bandage is not impeding circulation, press on a fingernail or toenail of the injured limb. If the nail quickly turns pink again, circulation is fine, and no adjustments are necessary. If the nail takes a minute or two to turn pink, or stays white, adjust the bandage as circulation is a problem. Keep doing the fingernail or toenail check as you remain with the person and adjust the bandage as needed.

## CPR or Cardiopulmonary Resuscitation

Cardiopulmonary Resuscitation or CPR is a technique used to stimulate the heart and lungs.

## When to Use CPR

Use CPR when the person's heart has stopped, or they are no longer breathing. CPR can also be used to help a person with distressed breathing—when they are gasping for breath.

## What is CPR

CPR involves us pushing down on a person's chest and assisting with breathing by blowing air into their mouths. We do this so that blood flows to the distressed person's brain and mechanically induces blood flow to other areas of the body, thus helping to prevent brain damage and death.

## Step-By-Step CPR

1. Check to see if the person is conscious.

If the person has no back or neck injury, gently shake or tap the person. Shaking someone with a spinal or head injury causes further injury. Shout "Are you okay?" If the person is not responding, move on to Step 2.

2. Start chest compressions.

For an adult or an older child who has reached puberty –

• Kneel next to the person.

• Using your fingers, locate the end of the breastbone where the ribs meet.

• Place two fingers at the tip of the breastbone.

• Place the heel of your other hand just above your fingers (pointing to the person's face).

• To compress the chest, use both hands. Remove your two fingers from the end of the breastbone and place them on top of the other hand. Then, lace your fingers and lift them so only the palms of your hands are in contact with the breastbone. 3. Position your arm and body for doing chest compressions by centering your shoulders directly above your hands on the person's chest.

3. Straighten your arms and lock your elbows. 4. In a steady rhythm, press down using your body weight. The force of each compression should go directly onto the breastbone, depressing it at least 2 in. (5 cm). Allow the chest to re-expand after each compression.

4. If you are not trained in CPR, give at least 100 chest compressions a minute. Push hard at about one to two times a second.

5. If you are trained in CPR, start Rescue Breaths. If you are not trained in CPR, don't worry about doing

Rescue Breaths, as chest compressions by themselves are effective on adults and older children. Children and babies benefit the most from rescue breathing.

6. Continue with 100 compressions a minute. Remember to allow time for the chest to expand, until the person is breathing normally.

7. If you are trained in CPR, give 30 compressions and two rescue breaths. Continue this cycle until help arrives or the person begins breathing normally.

8. When giving rescue breaths, check that the person's airway is not narrowed or blocked by an obstruction, including the tongue, during muscle relaxation. Remember to lift the chin and tilt the head back to allow rescue breaths to travel down the airway. Exhaled air contains only about five percent less oxygen than the air we breathe in. (Piazza, et al. 2014) This is enough oxygen to supply another person with oxygen, and forcing exhaled air into their lungs could possibly save their life. Rescue breathing also forces air into the person's air passages, the air sacs in their lungs, and so into the bloodstream and into red blood cells. By removing your mouth, the person's chest can fall, exhaling air with waste products.

9. Pocket masks can be used during CPR and may be available from a first aid kit or first aid station. However, CPR should never be delayed, even to find a pocket mask.

# Rescue Breaths

1. Place one hand on the person's forehead. 2. With your thumb and forefinger, pinch the person's nose closed.

2. Place the fingers of your free hand against the bone of the person's jaw and, if they have no neck injuries, tilt their chin up to ensure the airway is open.

3. Take a normal breath, seal your mouth over the person's mouth. If you are assisting with a baby, place your mouth over the baby's mouth and nose. Blow into the person's mouth for one second, then watch to see if their chest rises.

4. If their chest does not rise, tilt their chin back and give another rescue breath.

5. Between rescue breaths, remove your mouth from the person's face and breathe normally. Allow their chest to rise and fall and feel their exhale.

Special instructions for younger children

If a young child isn't breathing:

1. Kneel by their chest or head.

2. **Using only one hand**, apply compressions to the center of the chest, not directly onto their abdomen, end of their breastbone or ribs.

3. Give 30 compressions every minute, allowing for the expansion of the chest after every compression. Don't remove your hand during the expansion of the chest.

4. When checking their airway in the CPR position, don't sweep your finger in their mouth to clear it.

5. Call for help.

6. If you are trained in giving Rescue breaths, give two breaths after every 30 compressions.

7. Continue until help arrives.

Special instructions for infants

Always stand or kneel side-on to the infant when treating them. If the infant isn't breathing:

1. Never shake the baby to check the response. Call them and flick a finger gently at the sole of their feet.

2. Check that their airway is clear:

- Roll a towel and place it under their shoulders.

- Place a finger against their forehead and push it gently back.

- With one finger on the bony part of their chin, gently tilt their chin up. Avoid touching the soft tissue under their chin as this may cut off their airway.

3. CPR for infants:

- Check their airway is clear.

- Use two straightened fingers to deliver compressions to the center of their chest.

- Ensure you depress gently to about ⅓ of their chest capacity.

- Allow their chest to expand after every compression without removing your fingers.

- Give 30 compressions at a rate of 100 compressions a minute.

- Check their airway. Remove any visible objects. Don't sweep your finger in their mouth to clear out objects as it may deliver the object into their throats.

4. Hold the infant in the recovery position: cradle the baby with their head to the side lower than their torso.

Special instructions for Pregnant Women

When setting a pregnant woman on the ground to do the A-B-C, CPR or in the recovery position, elevate her right hip with tightly packed rolled-up towels or clothing if there is no one to help you.

When placing her in the recovery position, roll her onto her left side.

## The Heimlich Maneuver

You may have heard of this technique before. It is also called Abdominal Thrusts.

When to Use the Heimlich Maneuver

Use the Heimlich Maneuver when a person is choking.

How to Perform the Heimlich Maneuver

1. *Performing the Heimlich Maneuver on a person in distress -* 1. Stand behind the person, or kneel behind them if they are a child. Keep one of your feet slightly ahead of the other to balance yourself. Wrap your arms around their waist and tip the person slightly forward.

2. With one hand, make a fist and place it just above their navel.

3. With your other hand, grasp your fist. Press hard into their abdomen in a fast, upward motion as if you're trying to lift them off the ground.

4. Repeat the maneuver six to ten times until their airway is cleared of the blockage.

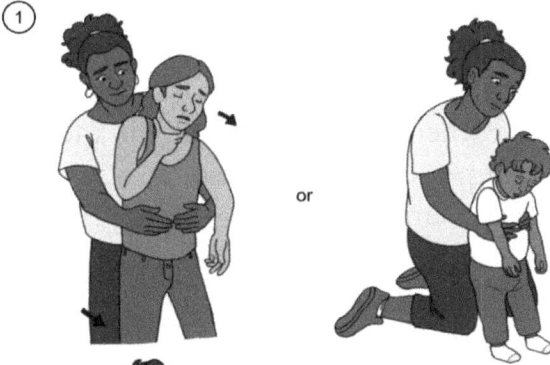

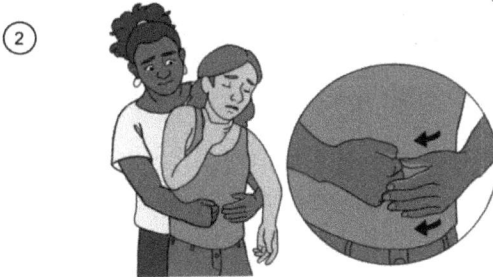

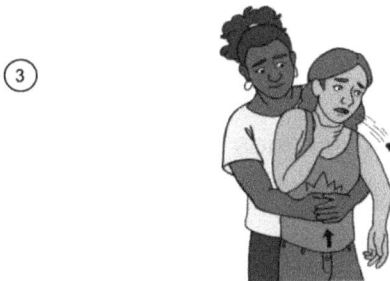

# Taking a Pulse (Heart Rate)

The rate at which your heart beats is called a pulse. A pulse can be felt in certain locations of the body where larger blood vessels are close to the skin's surface—areas such as your wrist and neck.

The standard pulse for an adult not exerting themselves is usually between 60 to 100 beats per minute. Your pulse may change in times of illness, so it is important to know your usual pulse when you are generally fit and healthy. To find your resting pulse or usual pulse, take your pulse only after you've been sitting or resting quietly for about five minutes. However, in the case of an emergency, a pulse should be taken immediately.

## How to Take Your Pulse

Check your pulse on the inside of your wrist.

- Place two fingers on the artery below your thumb to feel your pulse. Always use your fingers and never your thumb as your thumb has its own pulse that will make counting beats difficult.

- Use a light, gentle touch so you can detect even a light pulse.

- Count the beats for 30 seconds, then multiply by two to get the beats per minute—your pulse rate.

- You can also record if your pulse is strong or weak, and regular or irregular.

## How to Take Someone's Pulse

- For babies, take their brachial pulse by placing two fingers on the inner side of their upper arm. For older children, you can take their radial pulse at the wrist or their carotid pulse at the hollow of their neck and clavicle. Their pulse rate should be higher than a healthy adult's but still within the 60-100 beats per minute rate.

- For an adult, you can place two fingers on their wrist or their carotid artery on their neck to find their pulse. If the person is fit, their pulse rate may be slower.

## Splinting

A splint is used to prevent further injury to an arm, leg, fingers or toes that may be severely sprained, fractured, or broken by immobilizing it until professional help arrives. A splint may also be useful in the event of a snakebite while awaiting help.

## How to Splint a Limb

Use one of two methods -

1. Tie the injured arm or leg to a stiff, sturdy object. your aim is to prevent the limb bending, so any stiff object of a suitable length will do, such as a stick, a cane, or even rolled up magazines and newspapers. Use a belt, a rope, a bandage, or another suitable item to tie the splint securely to the limb. Ensure that the splint is not too tight and does not impede circulation and that it prevents any bending of the limb.

2. Secure the injured finger, toe, or limb to another part of the body. For example, you may tape an injured finger to the finger adjacent to it or fasten an injured arm so it is held against the chest. Ensure the splint is not too tight and is not causing further injury or discomfort to the person.

3. In the event of a fracture or snakebite, splinting is only an emergency measure. Professional health care must be sought immediately.

①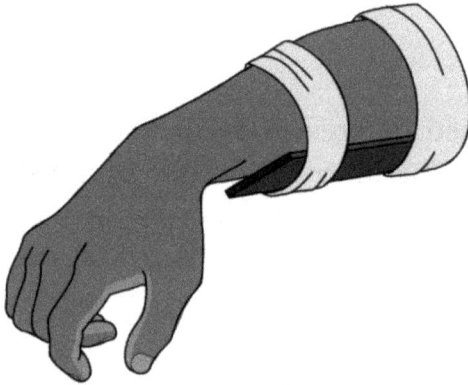

②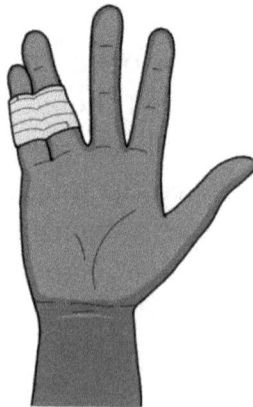

# Rules to Observe While Splinting

- Splint a limb from the joint above an injury to the joint below the injury. For example, splint a broken shin from above the knee to the ankle.

- If you have to transport the person a long or difficult distance, additional support to splints may be required.

- Never secure the splint directly over the injury, i.e. never tie ropes, belts or other fasteners directly over a fracture or snakebite.

- Always ensure that the splint, while securely fastened, never affects circulation. Do the fingernail test to check if circulation remains healthy.

- In some cases, swelling may occur over the injury. Adjust the splint by loosening it to ensure that circulation is not cut off.

- Always use padding when splinting knees and ankles if they are tied together.

# Slings

A sling is often used to immobilize an arm in the case of a suspected fracture (including rib fracture), dislocation, or other injuries. A sling's function is to hold the injured arm, bent at the elbow, comfortably across the person's torso. Usually, the hand of the bent arm, points upwards towards the opposite shoulder as the sling supports the weight of the forearm.

If no slings or triangular bandages are available, then a sling can be easily improvised using clothing for a short-term measure until medical help and a sturdier sling can be used.

Note: Once in a sling, it is important to regularly check circulation by noting the color of the person's fingernails (they should be healthy pink) and ensuring the person's arm doesn't begin to tingle or feel numb.

## Improvising Slings

- Use a jacket or button-up coat. Undo the button of a coat, waistcoat, or jacket around the person's chest. Slip in their arm, resting their wrist on the button beneath. Alternatively, use the corner of the jacket. Undo the jacket fastening. Fold the bottom end up and over the injured arm forming a cradle for the arm. Pin the edge of the jacket to the person's shoulder with safety pins. Tuck in any edges.

- If the person is using a long-sleeved shirt, position their injured arm across their chest with the elbow bent, pin the cuff of the shirt to their breast. Alternatively, pin their cuff to their shoulder if an elevated sling is needed.

- Use a belt, long, thin scarf, a tie, etc. to create a looped sling. Create a loop with the belt or scarf (tie or fasten the ends together) and hang it around the person's neck. Twist the lower end of the loop to create a lower loop (the item will now be in figure eight) and slip the person's hand through the lower-loop. Avoid this method if you suspect a wrist injury.

- Use a meter square of strong material or a large square scarf. Fold the material into a triangle (bring diagonally opposite ends together), and knot at the shoulder to form a cradle for the arm. Ensure the knot is safe and secure—square knots are best—and that the person's arm is comfortable. Tuck in the material ends by the elbow.

## Treating Convulsions and Fits

1. If the person is convulsing, lie them on their back in a safe place free of sharp and hard objects.

2. Turn the person onto their side so that their tongue moves to the front of the mouth and froth can freely flow out of their mouth.

3. Place a folded cloth under the person's head or hold their head so that they don't injure themselves from banging their head.

4. Allow the person to move their arms and legs, and to shake.

5. Loosen tight clothing.

6. Don't try to open the person's mouth or place anything in it.

## Handing Over to Paramedics

When paramedics or other professional medical personnel arrive:

- Continue assisting the person in distress until the paramedics ask you to step aside

- Tell the medical personnel all that you can, including details of the injury, your treatment, and details about medication

- Assist the paramedics further until they ask you to step aside

- Hand your notes to the paramedics

- Ensure all the person's belongings are in their care or that of the paramedic crew

# Chapter 3
# Mild Emergencies

Not all emergencies may be a risk to life, yet they can be overwhelming to deal with if you aren't sure how to treat them. Most common emergencies not requiring urgent medical attention occur at home, while traveling, during leisure activities—almost anywhere and at any time. Let's look at how to treat some common emergencies without calling for medical assistance from the outset.

## Bites and Stings

Almost everyone will experience bites and stings, particularly when outdoors and during spring and summer. Most bites and stings can be quickly and efficiently treated. However, stings in the mouth, throat or multiple stings must be medically treated as they obstruct the airways and are more likely to lead to anaphylaxis.

## What Not to Do

The following will cause infection and intensify the effects of the venom. You may also harm yourself in the process.

1. Don't cut into the wound or cut it out.

2. Don't attempt to suck venom out of a wound.

3. Don't use a tourniquet or tight bandage.

4. Don't treat the wound with chemicals or medicines (for example, potassium permanganate crystals) or inject them into the wound.

5. Don't put ice packs on the wound.

6. Don't use proprietary snake bite kits.

7. Applying traditional and herbal remedies on severe stings and bites may not be of much help and can even be life-threatening. It may be better to find professional medical assistance or hospitalization as soon as possible.

## General Rules to Treat Bites and Stings

Your priority: Keep the person calm and still, prevent rapid swelling, arrange transport and care to a medical facility.

1. Reassure and comfort the distressed person. Most people will panic when stung or bitten. In a calm voice, explain that most bites and stings from insects, spiders, snakes, and sea creatures are harmless, and even dangerous creatures seldom carry a poison that harms humans.

2. While keeping the person calm, keep them still with the injured body part below the level of the heart. Movement, particularly of an injured limb, and fear and excitement spread the venom quickly and worsen the person's condition. Consider using a splint to immobilize a bitten arm or leg.

3. Remove the person's rings, watch, bracelets, anklets, and shoes, and loosen restrictive clothing if there is swelling.

4. The patient should lie on one side in the recovery position to ensure their airway is clear and in case of fainting or vomiting.

5. Do not feed the person anything by mouth—food, alcohol, medicines, or drinks—unless there is a delay in

getting medical care or the risk of dehydration. Then, only allow the person water.

6. If the person has been stung in the mouth or throat, give them an ice cube to suck or let them sip ice water to reduce swelling and keep their airway open until help arrives.

7. Try to identify the animal that caused the wound, but don't attempt to capture or hold the creature if this may put you and others at risk. If the animal is dead, take it to the hospital with the person, but handle it with great care as even dead animals may still inject venom.

8. Arrange to transport the person to a hospital, a clinic, or another professional medical center as soon as possible. Ensure that the person remains as still as possible. Don't allow the person to walk. If no ambulance or other vehicle is available, carry them on a stretcher or a makeshift one. If a bicycle is available, carry them across the handlebar of the bike.

9. Antivenom, if available, should only be administered if there is evidence of severe poisoning, and in a location where resuscitation can be given, such as a medical center or hospital as the person may experience an allergic reaction. Antivenom must not be used if there are no signs of poisoning.

## Dog and Cat Bites

Cat and dog bites usually leave small puncture wounds. However, if there's a tearing of flesh, medical care must be sought.

## Treating Dog and Cat Bites

Your priority: Cleanse the wound, prevent inflammation and infection, and seek medical help if you suspect the animal is ill.

1. Wash the wound with water to remove the bacteria-rich saliva of the animal.

2. Keep the bitten area lower than the heart, if possible.

3. Bathe the wound in a mild solution of permanganate of potash.

4. Apply a clean dressing.

If you suspect the animal is rabid, seek medical help immediately.

# Spider Bites

Spider bites seldom cause major injury. However, venomous spiders such as black widow spider and the brown recluse spider can be quite dangerous.

### Seek immediate medical help when:

- The bite is from a black widow or brown recluse spider.
- You're not sure if the spider might be poisonous.
- The person has a growing ulcer at the site of the bite or severe abdominal cramping.
- The person isn't breathing.

### Treating Spider Bites

Your priority: Cleanse the wound. Prevent inflammation and infection.

1. Cleanse the wound using mild soap and water. Apply an antibiotic ointment.

2. If the bite is on an arm or leg, elevate the limb. Apply a cool compress to reduce pain and swelling. Dampen a cloth with cold water or fill the cloth with ice.

3. Over-the-counter pain medication can be used for further pain management, and, if the wound is itchy, an antihistamine (Benadryl, Chlor-Trimeton, etc.) may help.

4. A tetanus shot may be needed if the person bitten has not had one in five years.

## Snake Bites

Despite common perception, only about 15% of snakes worldwide are a danger to humans.

### Treating Snake Bites

Your priority: Seek medical help, move the person away from the snake, cleanse the bite.

While waiting for medical help:

1. Move out of the snake's striking distance.

2. Remain calm and still to prevent fast dispersion of the venom into the bloodstream.

3. Discard jewelry and tight clothing before swelling begins.

4. Position the person, if possible, so that the bite is below or at the level of the heart.

5. Cleanse the bite with soap and water.

6. Cover the bite with a clean, dry dressing.

**What Not to Do:**

- Don't apply ice or use a tourniquet.

- Don't attempt to remove the venom by cutting the wound or sucking on the bite.

- Don't allow the person bitten any caffeine or alcohol as these quickens the body's absorption of venoms.

- Don't attempt to capture the snake. Try to remember its color and shape, and other distinguishing features you can describe that will help in the identification for treatment. If you have your smartphone handy and it is safe to do so, take a photo of the snake for easier identification.

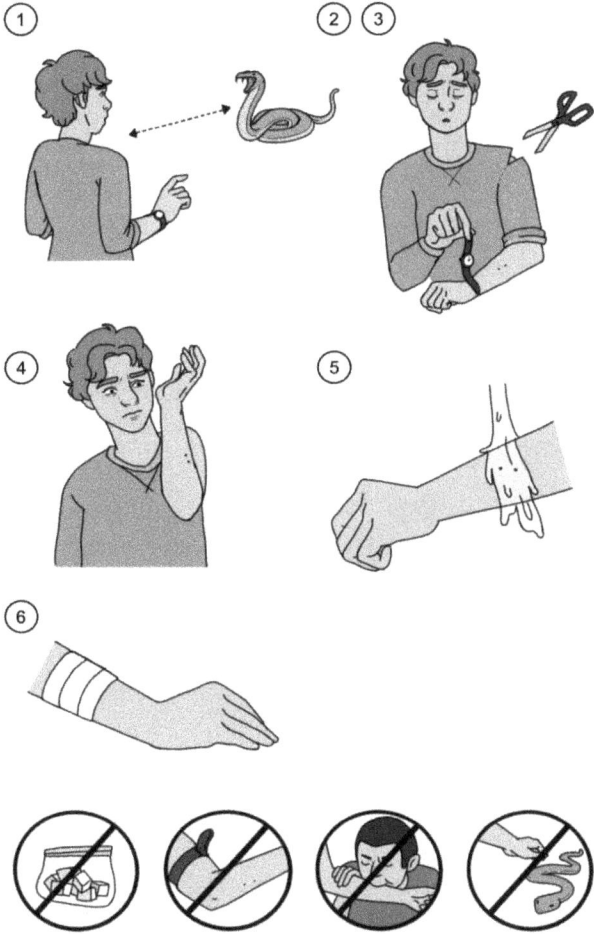

## Human Bites

Human bites can be even more dangerous than most animal bites as the human mouth contains vast amounts of bacteria and viruses. Human bites that break the skin can therefore become infected. When someone's knuckles are cut by another person's teeth (as may happen in a fight) this, too, is considered a human bite. When you do the same to yourself during a fall or accident, it is also considered a human bite.

**Treating Human Bites**

Your priority: Stop the bleeding. Seek medical care.

1. Stop bleeding by applying pressure with a clean, dry cloth.

2. Wash the wound thoroughly with soap and water.

3. Cover the wound with non-stick, clean bandage.

4. Seek medical care.

5. If the person bitten hasn't had a tetanus shot in five years, a booster shot may be needed within 48 hours of the bite.

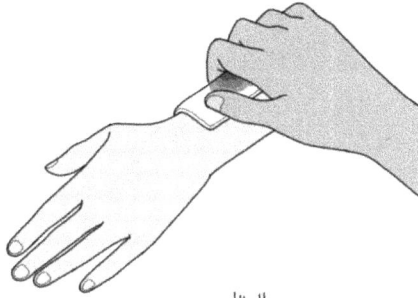

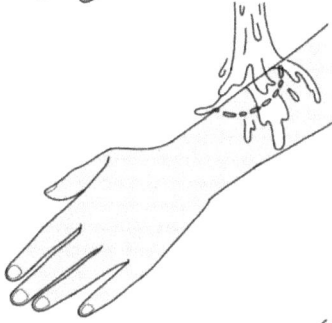

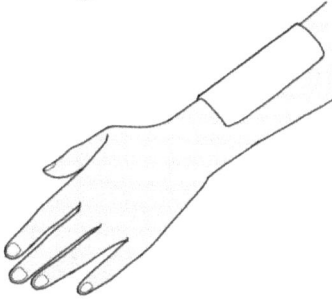

## Stings

Insect stings seldom cause major injury, but they can cause severe pain, particularly if the sting is on the lips or mouth.

### Treating Stings

Your priority: Remove the sting. Prevent inflammation and infection.

1. If a sting is from a bee, hornet, wasp, or similar insect, remove the thorny sting with a pair of tweezers. If no tweezers are available, apply pressure around the sting to force it up and out, or use a plastic card such as a credit card to scrape it off by scraping from the thorny side.

2. Wash the wound thoroughly with soap and water. If available, apply an ointment or lotion to relieve itching.

3. Caution the person not to scratch the sting as this can cause infection.

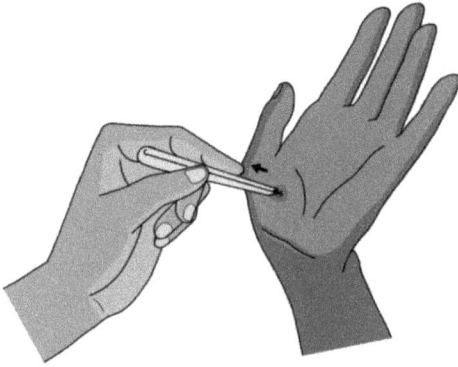

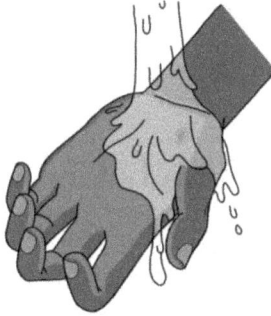

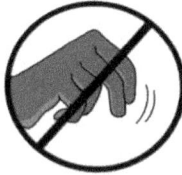

## Choking

A person chokes when an object obstructs their windpipe and interferes with their breathing, usually causing them a severe shortage of breath.

## Signs and Symptoms

- Most people will clutch their throat when choking
- An inability to talk
- Labored or noisy breathing
- Squeaky sounds when trying to breathe
- Coughing that's weak or forceful
- Skin, lips, or nails turning dusky or blue
- Flushed skin that soon turns pale or bluish
- Loss of consciousness

## Treating Someone Who Is Choking

Your priority: Dislodging the blockage as quickly as possible, assisting with breathing if necessary.

1. If the person can cough strongly, encourage them to cough the obstruction out.

2. Dislodge the object in their throat by leaning their head and shoulders forward and thumping their back hard between the shoulder blades. If a child is choking, hold them upside down and thump their backs between the shoulder blades.

3. If the person cannot cry, laugh hard, or talk, the American Red Cross recommends the Five-and-Five approach to assist the distressed person:

a) Thump the person's back 5 times.

b) Stand to the side and just behind a choking adult. If it is a child choking, kneel behind them. Place one hand across their chest for support. Bend the person's waist as you thump them between the shoulder blades with the heel of your hand.

c) Perform five Abdominal Thrusts, also known as the Heimlich Maneuver.

d) Alternate between five thrusts and five abdominal thrusts until the object is dislodged.

4. If you are alone and choking, you can perform abdominal thrusts on yourself by:

a) Placing your fist just above your navel.

b) Grasping your fist with your other hand and bending over a hard surface such as a desk, chair, or countertop.

c) Shoving your fist inward and upward.

5. To clear the airway of a pregnant or obese person:

a) During the Heimlich Maneuver, position your hands a little higher, just under the breastbone and the conjunction of the lowest ribs.

b) Perform the Heimlich Maneuver with a quick thrust.

c) Repeat until the object is dislodged from the throat.

6. If the person becomes unconscious. Perform the following steps.

a) Lower the person to the floor on their back with their arms to the side.

b) Clear the airway as in the A-B-C.

c) Begin <u>CPR</u> if the person remains unresponsive and the object remains lodged in their airway. The chest compressions may dislodge the obstruction.

d) Check the mouth often to ensure their airway remains clear and for the dislodged object.

7. To clear the airway of an infant who is not yet a year old:

a) Sit down. Hold the infant across your forearm. Rest your forearm on your thigh. Support the baby's head and neck with your hand and place their head lower than their trunk.

b) Using the heel of your hand, gently thump their back between the shoulder blades five times. Keep your fingers pointed up, so you don't hit the infant's head. Gravity and your blows combined should dislodge the object.

c) If the infant is still not breathing, turn the infant face-up on your forearm, supported by your thigh with their head lower than their trunk. Use two fingers placed on the center of their breastbone, give five quick compressions. Press down about 1.5 inches and allow the chest to rise in between compressions.

d) If breathing doesn't resume, repeat the back blows and chest compressions. Call for medical help.

e) Do <u>Infant CPR</u> if the object dislodges but the infant doesn't begin breathing.

8. If the child is older than a year old and conscious, administer the <u>Heimlich Maneuver</u>, taking care not to use too much force as this can injure the child's ribs and internal organs.

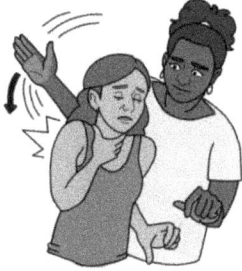

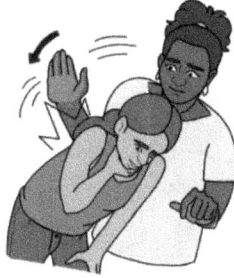

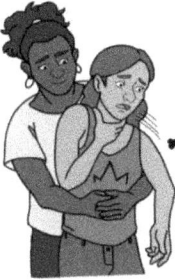

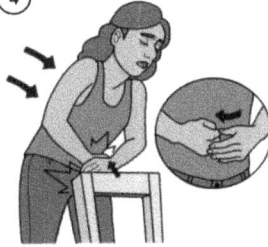

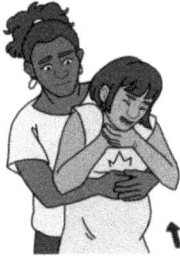

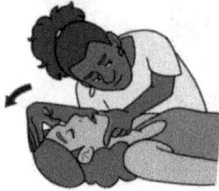
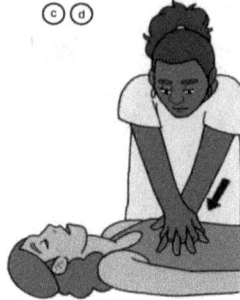

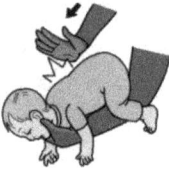
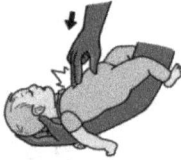
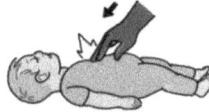

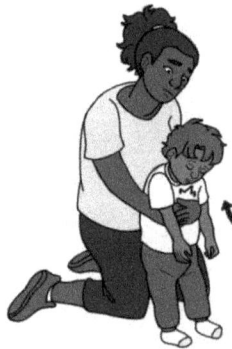

## Eye Trauma

When foreign bodies enter the eye, they can cause discomfort in the eyeball and eyelid. If the foreign body becomes embedded in the eyeball, it can cause severe problems.

## Treating Eye Trauma

Your priority: Prevent further injury to the eye, remove irritants safely, promote recovery of the eye.

1. Prevent the person from rubbing their eye. Position them so that they are facing your light and you can stand in front of them.

2. Pull down their lower eyelid. With the corner of a clean cloth or handkerchief (white, twirled up, and moistened, if possible) remove the foreign object.

3. If the object is embedded, don't attempt to remove the object. Have the person close their eye and apply a soft pad of cotton wool secured with a bandage.

4. If the foreign body is not found and you suspect that it lies under the upper eyelid, encourage the person to blink underwater. Alternatively, lift the upper eyelid forward, push the lower lid below it and release both lids simultaneously. The lower lid lashes may brush out the object from the upper eyelid.

5. If a liquid irritant is in the eye, get the person to blink underwater or flush the eyes out with copious amounts of water. Apply a soft cotton pad over the eye kept in position by a pair of shades or a lightly fixed bandage.

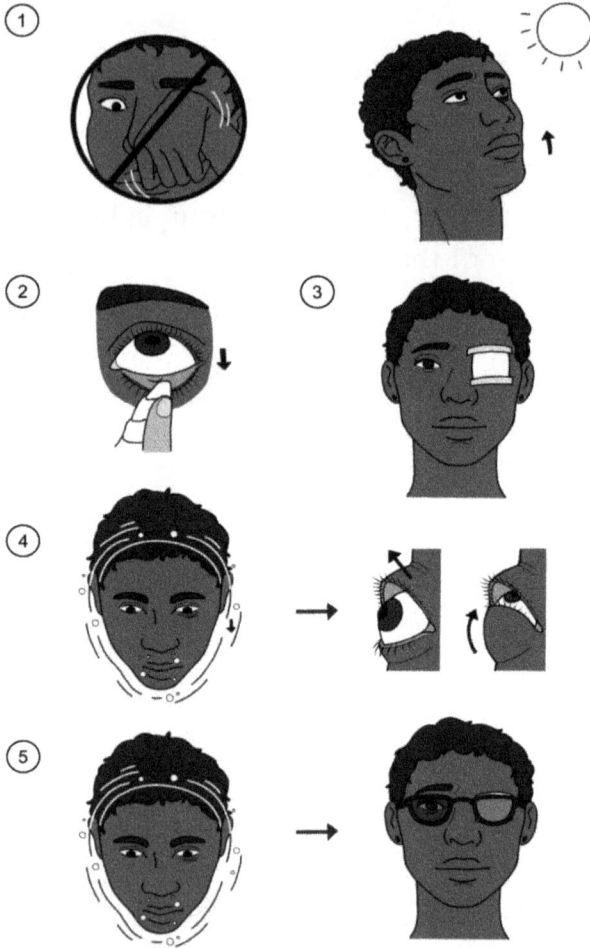

## Nosebleed

A common emergency in anyone of any age, nosebleeds are usually not a true medical problem, but can sometimes indicate a severe problem.

# Treating Nosebleeds

Your priority: Stop the nosebleed by pinching the nostrils shut.

1. Sit the person down and lean their head forward to reduce blood pressure in the nose and to discourage further bleeding. This position prevents them from swallowing blood which can cause stomach irritation.

2. Get the person to gently blow their nose to clear blood clots in their nose. Spray both sides of the nose with a nasal decongestant with oxymetazoline (Afrin).

3. Pinch their nostrils shut using your thumb and forefinger. Instruct them to breathe through their mouth. Keep their nose pinched shut for about 10 to 15 minutes. This often stops the bleeding as it puts pressure on the point of the nose that is bleeding.

4. If the nosebleed persists after 10 to 15 minutes, continue pinching their nose shut for another 10 to 15 minutes. Avoid looking into the nose. If the bleeding still hasn't stopped, get emergency medical care.

5. Advise the person with the nosebleed to avoid blowing or picking their nose, and avoid bending down, for several hours. Keep their head higher than their heart. If available, apply petroleum jelly gently into the nostrils using a cotton swab or a finger.

6. If the bleed resumes, repeat the steps above, but if the nosebleed persists, get medical care as soon as possible.

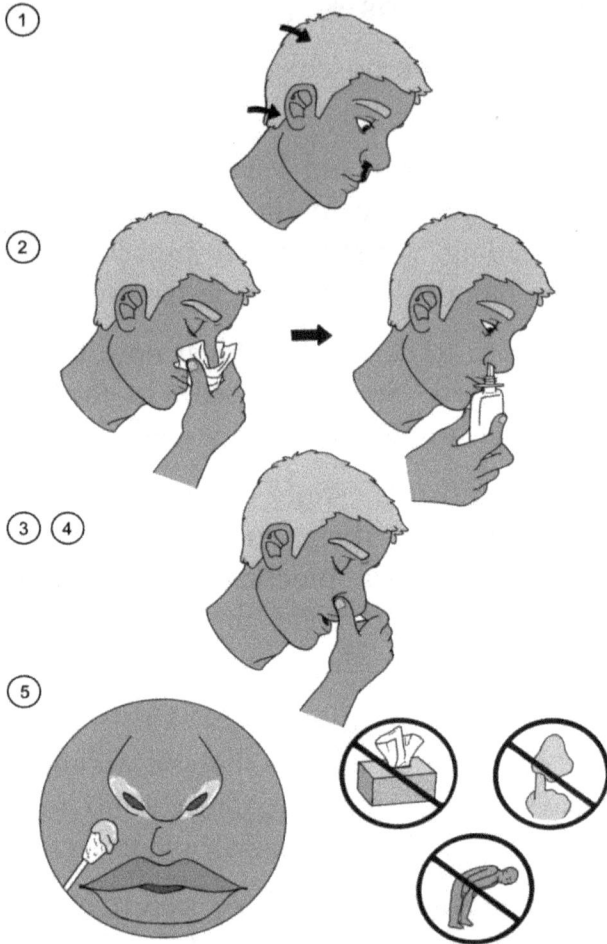

## Fainting

Fainting occurs when a person's brain experiences a temporary shortage of blood resulting in a brief loss of consciousness. A faint can have little medical significance, or it can be an indicator of a serious medical condition, usually involving the heart.

## Treating Fainting

Your priority: Keeping the person still and out of danger. Assist with breathing if necessary.

If you feel faint:

1. Lie down or sit down.

2. If you're sitting down, place your head between your legs for a minute or two.

3. Avoid fainting again by slowly and cautiously getting up. Keep your movements slow.

4. If someone else faints:

5. Set the person on their back.

6. Loosen restrictive clothing such as ties, scarfs, collars, and belts.

7. If they aren't injured and they're breathing, raise their legs above their heart level—about 12 inches or 30 centimeters.

8. Don't allow the person to get up quickly or too soon to avoid them fainting again.

9. Check the person's breathing. If they stop breathing, perform CPR.

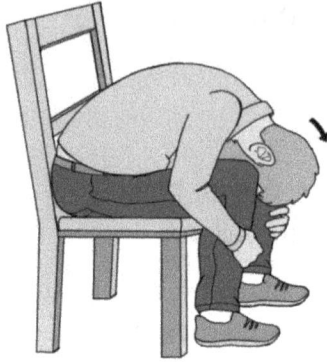

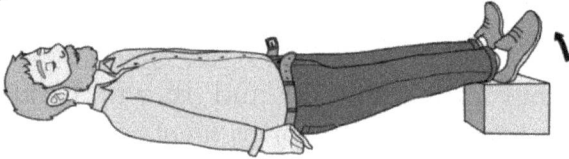

## Headaches

Most headaches are minor emergencies and don't require medical attention. However, sometimes a headache can indicate quite serious conditions. Serious or dangerous headaches are often unexplained and persistent. Get medical advice or care as soon as possible in those cases.

Headaches can be treated with pain relievers. Alternative remedies are also possible treatments. Consult

## Migraines

Migraines are quite common, particularly in women.

## Signs and Symptoms of Migraines

- Causes moderate to severe pain, stemming from one or more triggers
- Pulsates or throbs
- Causes nausea, vomiting, increases sensitivity to light and sound.
- Usually affects one side of the head but can affect both sides.
- Worsens with activity such as climbing steps
- Lasts four to 72 hours without treatment

## Treating Migraines

The aim of treating a migraine is to alleviate the symptoms and avoid extending the migraine attack.

If migraine triggers are known, migraine management and avoiding or alleviating triggers is crucial to reduce the severity and duration of a migraine. Treatment may take various forms or combinations of individual treatments.

Treatments may include:

- Rest in a quiet, dark room
- Applying hot or cold compresses to the back of the head or neck.

- Massage and small amounts of caffeine if the person is not a heavy coffee drinker.

- Over-the-counter painkillers such as ibuprofen (Advil, Motrin, etc.), aspirin (if the person isn't on blood thinning medication or allergic to it), and acetaminophen (Tylenol and others).

- Preventive and prescription medication such as metoprolol (Lopressor), propranolol (Innopran, Inderal, etc., amitriptyline, divalproex (Depakote), topiramate (Qudexy XR, Trokendi XR, Topamax, erenumab-aooe (Aimovig)

## Foodborne Illness

Foodborne illness often occurs when the natural bacteria in all food multiplies excessively when food is not cooked, cleaned, or stored properly. Food can also be contaminated by chemicals, toxins, viruses, and parasites.

## Signs and Symptoms

- Diarrhea, often turning bloody
- Nausea
- Abdominal pain
- Vomiting
- Dehydration
- Low-grade fever at times

Excessive dehydration can result in further symptoms:

- Feeling faint or light-headed, particularly when upright
- Tiredness

- Dark-colored urine
- Less frequent urination
- Excessive thirst

## Treating Foodborne Illnesses

Your priority: Ensure the person is hydrated.

1. Let the person slowly sip liquids (water or sports drinks with electrolytes). This prevents dehydration and sipping, instead of ingesting large amounts of liquids at once, and prevents vomiting and nausea.

2. Look for signs of dehydration. Monitor urination. Infrequent and dark urine instead of frequent clear urine indicates dehydration. Feeling faint and dizzy are also signs of dehydration. If these signs appear despite hydrating as best you can, seek medical attention.

3. Anti-diarrheal medication must be avoided as they prevent or slow the cause of the diarrhea (organisms or toxins) being expelled from the body. You may want to check with a doctor if you are unsure how to proceed.

## Foreign Objects in the Nose

A foreign object in the nose can be very painful.

## Removing a Foreign Object from a Nose

Your priority: Avoiding further injury to the nose while gently coaxing out the object without force.

1. Don't probe for the object in the nose with a cotton swab.

2. Ask the person to not inhale the object any further, and to breathe through the mouth until their nose is clear.

3. Instruct them to blow their nose gently and calmly, without force and not in quick succession. If only one nostril is affected by the object, instruct the person to hold their clear nostril shut and commence breathing gently and calmly.

4. When the object is visible and may be easily reached and gripped by tweezers, gently remove the foreign object. Never attempt to remove an object you cannot see.

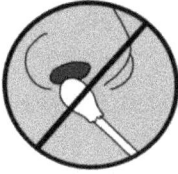
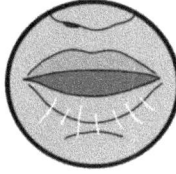
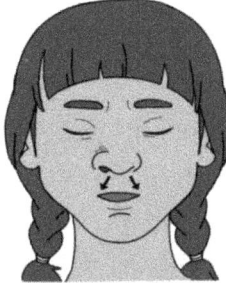
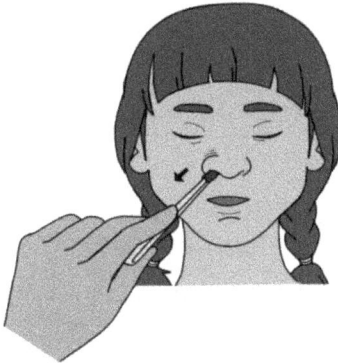

## Foreign Object in the Ear

A foreign object in the ear is not only painful, but can also cause a loss of hearing and infection.

### Removing a Foreign Object from an Ear

Your priority: Avoiding further injury and coaxing the object out of the ear by one of the following methods.

1. Avoid probing the ear with a cotton swab or other tool as you may push the object further into the ear canal and risk injury to the person.

2. If the object can be easily seen, easily reached and gripped with tweezers, and is pliant, gently remove it.

3. If the object cannot be seen, utilize gravity. Tip the person's head to the side with the affected ear pointing to the ground. Allow the object to fall out, if possible.

4. If the foreign object is an insect, use warm (not hot) oil to float the insect out of the ear by tilting the person's head with the affected ear facing up towards the light. Use baby oil, olive oil, or mineral oil. Only use this method to remove insects from the ears. If you suspect the person's eardrum may be perforated or you are assisting a child with ear tubes, don't use this method. Signs of a perforated eardrum include bleeding, pain, and a discharge from the ear.

5. Irrigate the ear with warm water using a bulb syringe to wash the object out of the ear. Don't use this method if the person has ear tubes in place or you suspect they may have a perforated eardrum.

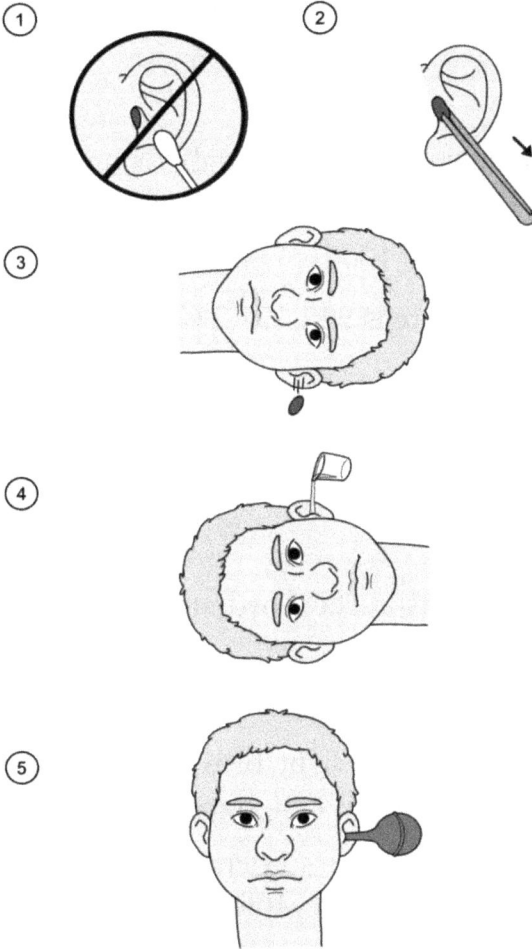

# Fever

When our body temperature rises above 100.4 F or 38 C, we have a fever. Fevers are often a sign of infection and most fevers we experience are not harmful. In many cases, they are helpful in fighting off an infection. Most fevers don't require medical treatment. However, some fevers over an extended period can be debilitating, or even fatal if no medical care is given. It is therefore wise to monitor fevers.

How to Check for a Fever:

- Internal temperature (ear, rectal, or temporal artery temperature) is 100.4 F (38 C) or higher.
- Oral temperature is 100 F (37.8 C) or higher.
- Armpit temperature is 99 F (37.2 C) or higher.

## Treating Fevers

Your goal is to promote rest and relieve discomfort.

For adults:

1. Ensure the person stays hydrated by drinking plenty of liquids.
2. Encourage them to dress in lightweight clothing.
3. Cover them with a light blanket if they experience chills. Once the chills end, remove the blanket.
4. Take acetaminophen (Tylenol, etc.) or ibuprofen (Advil, etc). Always follow the recommended dosage.
5. For children:
6. Ensure the child drinks plenty of liquids.
7. Encourage them to wear lightweight clothing.
8. If the child experiences the chills, cover them with a light blanket.
9. Never give aspirin to children or teens.
10. Don't give infants pain relievers.

**11.** If the child is 6 months or older, give them a child's dosage of acetaminophen (Tylenol, etc.) or ibuprofen (Advil, etc.). Always read the instructions and dosage before administering the medication.

For Adults:

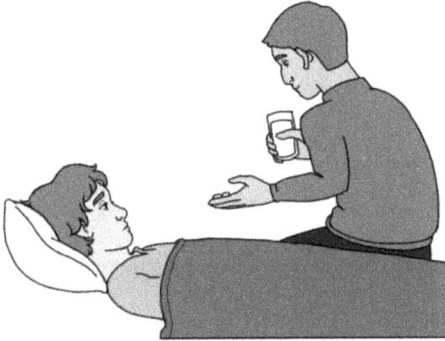

For Children:

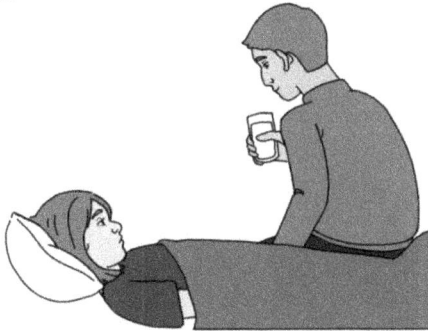

# Sunburn

We've all experienced sunburn after prolonged exposure to the sun. Sunburnt skin turns red, is painful and swollen.

Sometimes, blisters may appear. Headaches, fever, and nausea often accompany sunburn.

## Treat Sunburn

Your priority: Cool the skin, apply a soothing gel or cream, and hydrate the person.

1. Cool the skin by bathing in cool water or applying a cool compress by wetting a clean, soft towel in cold water.

2. Apply a moisturizer, gel, or lotion preferably containing calamine or aloe vera, both of which soothe the skin.

3. Ensure the person drinks plenty of water to stay hydrated.

4. Don't break any blisters that may form. If blisters burst, cleanse the skin gently with mild soap and water. Apply an antibiotic ointment. Cover the area with a non-stick gauze bandage. Should a rash develop, stop using the ointment and seek medical care.

5. Pain relievers such as ibuprofen (Advil, Motrin, IB, etc.) may be taken and may ease swelling. Other pain-relieving medications for sunburn may take the form of gels.

6. Keep the person out of the sun as their skin heals.

7. Apply an over-the-counter hydrocortisone cream for severe sunburn.

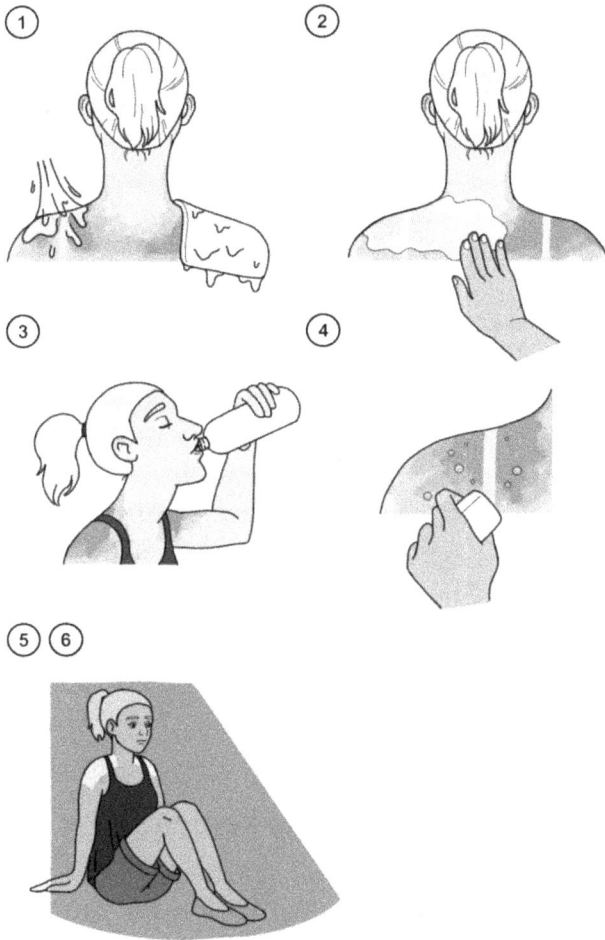

## Gastroenteritis

Gastroenteritis occurs when your intestines and stomach become inflamed. Symptoms can last from a day to more than a week, depending on the cause of the inflammation. Viruses and contaminated food or water are the most common causes of gastroenteritis. Side effects from a medication is another common cause of this illness.

Signs and Symptoms of Gastroenteritis:

- Nausea or vomiting
- Cramps
- Diarrhea
- Low grade fever in some cases

## Treating Gastroenteritis

Your priority: Ensure the person is hydrated. Monitor their condition.

1. To avoid dehydration, ensure the person drinks lots of liquids, particularly water, sports drinks, and other electrolyte replacement drinks. Encourage them to sip the liquids for some time as ingesting large amounts of liquids all at once may cause vomiting and nausea.

2. Monitor urination to guard against dehydration. The person should frequently be urinating with light to clear urine. Dark urine passed infrequently is a major sign of dehydration. Ask the person if they feel light-headed or dizzy. These are also signs of dehydration. If these signs appear despite their hydrating well, seek medical attention.

3. Slowly introduce small amounts of bland, easy to digest food. Encourage the person to eat small portions frequently to avoid nausea. Offer foods such as soda crackers, toast, gelatin, bananas, applesauce, rice, and chicken. If the person experiences nausea once again, stop serving food and resume the liquids. Alcohol, dairy, caffeine,

nicotine, fatty foods, and spicy food are to be avoided for a few days.

4. Encourage the person to rest as their bodies will be depleted and they will experience fatigue.

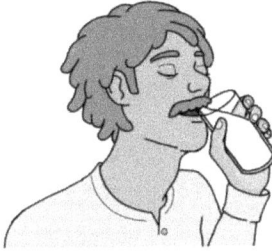

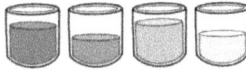

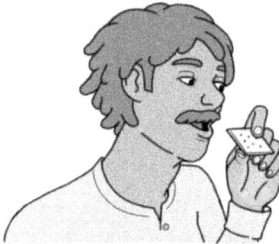

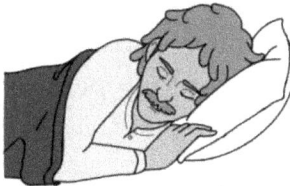

# Sprains

Between your joints lie ligaments, elastic-like structures that connect and allow the bones to work together. When the fibers of a ligament are torn in an injury, we call it a sprain.

The most common type of sprain is an ankle sprain. Knee, wrist, and thumb sprains are also common.

Signs of a sprain include rapid swelling and pain and difficulty moving the joint.

## Treating Sprains

Your priority: Keeping the person's weight off the limb and preventing swelling by icing the sprain.

1.  Keep the person's weight off their limb and rest the limb for at least 48 to 72 hours. This may mean the person must use a crutch, a splint, or a brace. However, activity should not be avoided.

2.  Apply ice or a cold compress to limit swelling. A slush bath, cold pack, or a compression sleeve filled with cold water can be used. Ice the injury as soon as possible for at least 15 to 20 minutes. During the next 48 to 72 hours, periodically ice the injury four to eight times a day until the swelling subsides. When using ice, be careful not to use it for long periods as this causes tissue damage.

Sprains can take days to months to recover. Once the pain and swelling subside, encourage the person to use the limb gently and with caution. They should experience gradual progress. However, care must be taken not to overtax the injured area and cause a repeat sprain.

# Hyperventilation

Hyperventilation is rapid breathing, often quite deep breathing which results in too little carbon dioxide in the body. This may lead to dizziness, tingling of the limbs, excessive sweating, and trembling. The person's pulse rate will also be very high.

Hyperventilation usually accompanies panic attacks but can also be the result of a medical condition, and emotional upset. Most children tend to hyperventilate due to emotional upset or a medical condition.

## Treating Hyperventilation

Your priority: Calming the person down. Helping them seek medical advice.

1. Speak firmly and kindly to the person.
2. Remove them from the upset or lead them to a quiet, open space.
3. Coach them to take slower breaths. If it helps, ask them to sit with their head between their knees for a minute or two.
4. Do not allow the person to breathe into a paper bag and rebreathe their expelled air as it could cause more harm if they have an infection.

# Chapter 4
# Serious Emergencies

Serious emergencies require swift attention. You will now learn the necessary actions to deal rapidly with unexpected emergencies that include shock, burns, cuts, and wounds. You will also learn to attend to various outdoor emergencies such as heat stroke, hypothermia, frostbite, fractures, and even electrocution. Remember, the less you panic and follow the steps in order, the more likely the situation will remain manageable until help arrives.

NB! Take care with the medications you give a distressed person. You are not allowed to give your own prescription medications or even direct someone else to go to a pharmacy to procure your own preference of a medication to be administered. Only use medication from a first aid kit in their recommended dosage.

## Shock

Shock is an indicator that a person's body is shutting down functions. This happens when your body cannot send enough blood to vital organs like the heart and brain.

Shock can be caused by a sudden injury, illness, bleeding, and even emotional distress. Mild injury can also cause shock.

## Symptoms of Shock

Adults and children may show the following symptoms:

- Fainting or falling unconscious
- Feeling faint, dizzy, or extremely light-headed

- Feeling very weak and losing motor-control, such as having trouble standing.

- Lack of alertness or feeling that they cannot think clearly. This may appear as confusion, fear, restlessness, or being unresponsive to questions.

Babies and younger children may show the following symptoms:

- Losing consciousness or passing out

- Extreme sleepiness or they are hard to wake up

- Unresponsive to touch or talk

- Hyperventilating

- Confusion. They may be unaware of their surroundings or unable to express where they are.

## Treating Shock

Your priority: Treat any bleeding, assist with breathing if necessary, ensure the person is warm and reassured.

1. Act promptly as this could save their life.

2. Get the person to lie down. In the event of a head, neck, or chest injury, keep their legs flat. If there is no such injury, raise their legs about 12 inches or 30 centimeters.

3. If the person vomits, roll them onto their side to drain their mouth. If you suspect the person has a chest, neck or head injury, gently roll their head, neck, shoulders and body together as a unit using the log roll technique from the A-B-C.

4. Stop any bleeding.

5. Splint any broken bones.

6. Ensure the person is warm, but not hot. In a cold environment, put a blanket under them and cover them with another blanket or a sheet. In a hot environment, keep the person cool and shaded from the sun.

7. Take the person's pulse.

8. Keep the person calm until they recover, or medical help arrives.

① ②

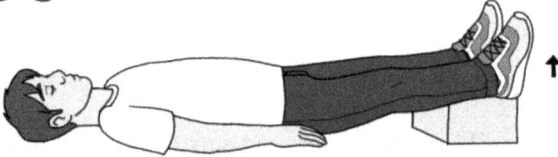

③

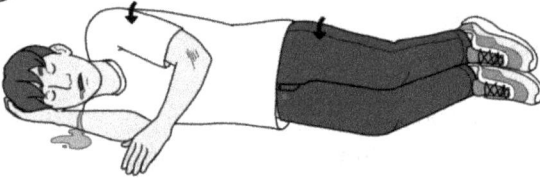

④ 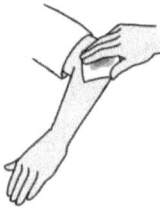 ⑤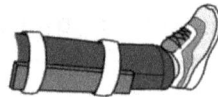

⑥ ⑦

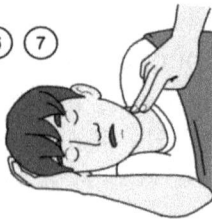

# Smoke Inhalation

If a person has inhaled smoke or fumes, they will have little oxygen in their body and may need help breathing. Besides smoke, most fires release toxic fumes from burnt plastics and other items, causing more respiratory problems and even poisoning.

If someone has passed out from fumes or smoke in an enclosed area, don't attempt to rescue them without first using appropriate breathing gear as you will most likely be overcome by the smoke or fumes yourself.

If a person is in a garage with a vehicle engine running, they will most likely have carbon monoxide poisoning. Open the garage first before attempting to help them.

Signs and Symptoms of Smoke and Fumes Inhalation:

- Coughing
- Hoarse breathing and shortness of breath
- Smarting and red, irritated eyes
- Tightness in chest and chest pains
- Headache
- Drowsiness and confusion
- Irregular or rapid pulse
- Soot in the mouth and nose
- Burns on skin or skin has a bluish tinge
- Nausea or vomiting (particularly with carbon monoxide poisoning)

## Treating Smoke Inhalation

Your priority: Call emergency services, help the person to find oxygen and breathe normally.

1. Call emergency services, telling them the nature of the fire or the fumes.

2. If it's safe for you to do so, help the person into an area away from the fire or fumes where there is clean air.

3. If their clothes are on fire, have them drop and roll on the ground.

4. If the person loses consciousness and stops breathing, give CPR.

5. Coach the person to breathe normally.

6. Treat any burns.

7. Stay with the person until medical help arrives. Anyone who experiences smoke inhalation must be treated by a doctor as some effects can persist for days, even months, and symptoms can be delayed.

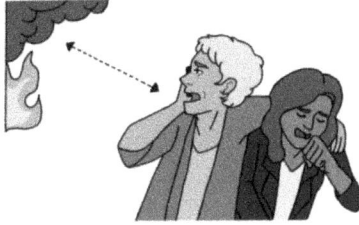

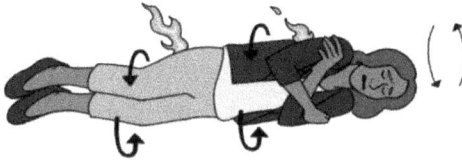

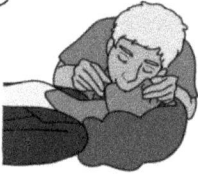

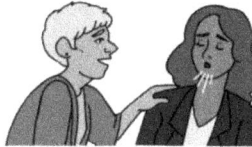

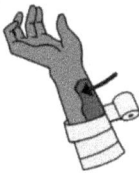

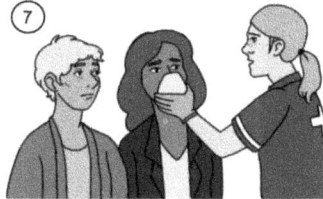

## Common and Chemical Burns and Scalds

Most burns, whether sustained at work or at home, tend to be minor injuries. When burnt by a hair appliance, hot stove, or hot water, home treatment is sufficient to treat the burn to avoid infection and promote healing.

Less common burns can result from dry heat such as hot metal, fire, contact with highly charged electrical current or friction from fast moving items such as rope or cloth. Burns can also result from mechanical devices such as revolving wheels, and corrosive chemicals that are strong acids or alkali.

A scald occurs when a person is injured by moist heat such as hot water, steam, hot oil, or tar.

## Types of Burns

Heat or thermal burns are caused by hot objects, hot liquids, fire, or steam. Scald burns from hot liquids and steam are the most common type of burn.

Cold temperature burns are caused when exposed skin is damaged by wet, windy, or cold conditions.

Electrical burns are caused when a person is harmed by contact with electrical sources or lightning.

Chemical burns are caused by contact with household or industrial chemicals in a liquid, gas, or solid form. Natural foods, such as chili peppers, contain substances that cause skin irritation and a burning sensation.

Radiation burns are caused by the sun, sunlamps, tanning booths, X-rays, or radiation treatment for cancer.

Friction burns result from friction from hard surfaces such as roads (road rash), carpets, or gym floors. These tend to be a combination of a scrape and a heat burn, Athletes may experience friction burns from floors, courts, or tracks when they fall. Bicycle and motorcycle riders without protective clothing may experience friction burns if they fall.

## Effects and Signs

Scalds and burns have the same effect. This may range from a reddening of the skin, blistering, destruction of the skin, and deeper tissue damage.

## Burn Degrees

The seriousness of a burn depends on its depth (damage to skin and inner tissue) and the size of the area burnt.

- First degree burns harm only the first layer of skin.

- Second degree burns fall into two categories:

  1. Superficial partial-thickness burns injure the first and second layers of skin.

  2. Deep partial thickness burns damage deeper layers of skin.

- Third degree burns damage all the layers of the skin as well as the tissue beneath. These burns must receive professional medical care.

- Fourth degree burns cause extensive damage to the body and must receive medical care. They may injure nerves, blood vessels, muscles, tendons, ligaments, and bones.

## Treating Thermal Burns

Burns sterilize the areas injured as well as the clothes worn in the affected area for a short period. Try to preserve their sterile nature for as long as possible.

Your main goal is to cool the skin down using cool, running water for 20 minutes, then assess the burn and the state of the distressed person. If no water is available. Follow the steps below.

1. Wash and sterilize your hands before assisting the person and handling the wound. Minimize handling of the wounded area.

2. Don't apply any lotions.

3. Don't remove clothing.

4. Don't break blisters.

5. Cover the affected area, including the burnt clothing, with a dry sterile dressing where possible. Clean lint or freshly laundered linen can also be used if no dressing is available.

6. When no blisters are present, bandage firmly. If blisters are present or suspected, bandage lightly.

7. Immobilize the affected area.

8. Treat the person for shock.

## Treating Chemical Burns

Your priority: Flush out the chemical with a neutralizing agent and water.

### For acids
1. Flush the affected area with water.

2. Bathe the affected area with copious amounts of an alkaline solution made from two teaspoons of baking soda or washing soda in one pint of warm water.

### For Alkalis
1. If the burn is a result of quicklime, brush any residue off.

2. Bathe the affected area with copious amounts of a weak acid solution made from vinegar or lemon juice diluted in an equal amount of warm water.

# Cuts and Wounds

## Types of Cuts and Wounds

- Incised wounds are caused by sharp instruments such as a razor or metal vegetable peelers.

- Lacerated wounds are noted by their torn and irregular edges and are often caused by machinery, animal claws, kitchen graters, etc.

- Contused wounds are caused by a direct blow or crushing and are often accompanied by bruising in the affected area.

- Puncture wounds are caused by a stab from sharp, pointed instruments such as needles, knives, and bayonets. Though they may have quite small visible wounds, the instrument may penetrate quite deeply.

## Treating Cuts and Wounds

Your priority: Reduce or stop bleeding, clean the wound, and pack or bandage the wound to prevent further opening of the wound.

1. Unless the person has a fracture, position them so that the wound is elevated.

2. Staunch the bleeding as much as possible before cleaning the wound. To stop the bleeding or staunch it, apply direct, steady pressure to the elevated wound for a full 15 minutes. Use a clock or timer to ensure a full 15

minutes have passed before checking to see if bleeding is under control. Resist checking the wound before then. If blood fully saturates the cloth over the wound, add another cloth or gauze pad over the first one without disturbing it. If there's an object in the wound, don't apply direct pressure on the object; apply pressure around the object.

3. Don't disturb any blood clots that are forming.

4. Remove as little clothing as possible and expose the wound. Jewelry in the area of the wound should also be removed so that if swelling occurs, the jewelry doesn't impede blood flow.

5. Remove foreign bodies that can be easily wiped off with a clean dressing or which can be easily picked out without disturbing the wound.

6. Apply a clean bandage or dressing.

7. Immobilize the injury. If the injury is by a joint, use a splint if necessary.

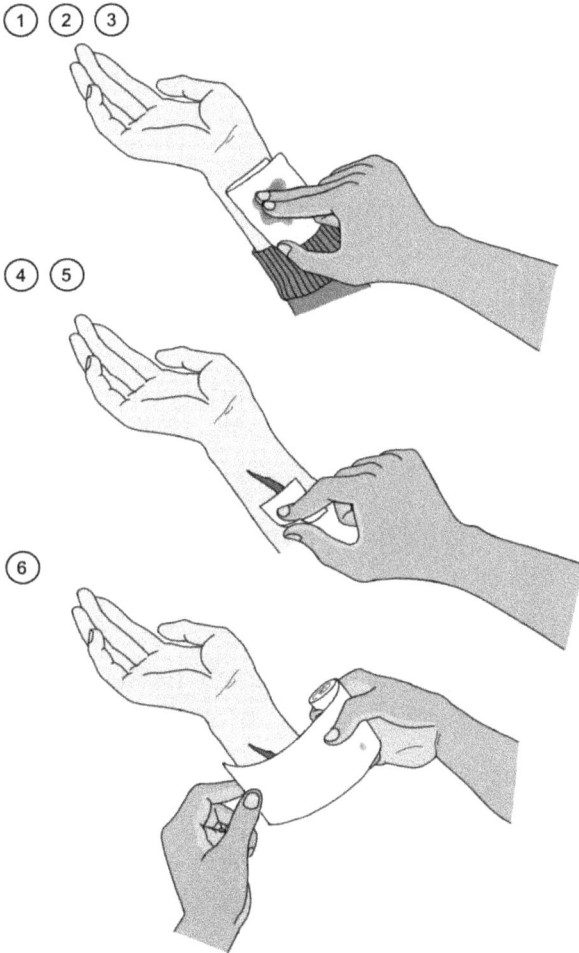

## Keep in Mind

- Mild bleeding usually stops or slows to a trickle after direct pressure is applied for 15 minutes. Sometimes, mild bleeding may still ooze for up to 45 minutes.

- If moderate to severe bleeding doesn't slow after 15 minutes of direct pressure, call for medical help while continuing to apply direct pressure to the wound.

- Don't use a tourniquet to stop bleeding.

- Clean the wound and do all you can to avoid further injury as well.

- If a foreign object is embedded in the wound and it cannot be easily removed, cover the object with a dressing. Stack sufficient pads around the wound without applying pressure to the object.

- If the cut is deep and there are no foreign objects present, ensure you pack padding into the wound's depths, and make sure you have sufficient pads at the skin level to apply pressure on ruptured blood vessels.

- While attending to the wound, monitor the person for signs of shock.

- Don't allow the person anything to eat or drink if their wound is severe as they may need an anesthetic. Moisten their lips with water if they are thirsty.

- While waiting for help, cover the person with a blanket if they are cold. Don't use a direct source of heat, such as a heat lamp to warm a severely wounded person.

## Severed Finger or Toe

Severed fingers or toes can result from vehicles and machinery—workplaces or in the garden—or accidents involving knives and other sharp recreational equipment. A finger or toe can be reattached to a hand or foot if care is taken from the outset. In the event of a cut or wound involving a severed finger or toe, follow these steps:

1. If machinery or a vehicle is involved, turn it off.

2. Call emergency services or arrange transportation of the person to a trauma unit.

3. If others can assist, ask them to locate the appendage if it has been amputated, and follow the steps from 11-16. If there is no one to help, locate the finger or toe after you have stopped the bleeding.

4. Without removing any clothing or jewelry from the injured hand or foot, elevate the injured limb.

5. Cleanse the wound with a saline solution.

6. Cover the injury with a sterile gauze or similar dressing.

7. Don't squeeze the wound or apply too much pressure on it as this causes further damage. Apply a light bandage if needed, and ensure circulation is good.

8. If the wound is still bleeding heavily, apply *light* pressure.

9. Treat the person for <u>shock</u>.

10. Don't allow the person any food or drink as they will be given an anesthetic at the hospital.

11. Once the amputated finger or toe is found, don't scrub it but wash it gently with a sterile saline solution.

12. Dampen a gauze dressing and wrap the appendage in it.

13. Place the finger or toe in a waterproof, clean, sealed plastic bag.

14. Into a larger plastic sealable bag, place the bag with the appendage.

15. Set the bundle on ice or surround it with ice or cold water in a cooler. Never place the severed finger or toe directly onto ice or cold water as this causes further damage.

16. If more than one finger or toe was severed right off, wrap them individually and seal in separate plastic bags to ensure the best outcome.

17. Ensure the severed appendages always travel with the person to the trauma unit so there is no delay in surgery.

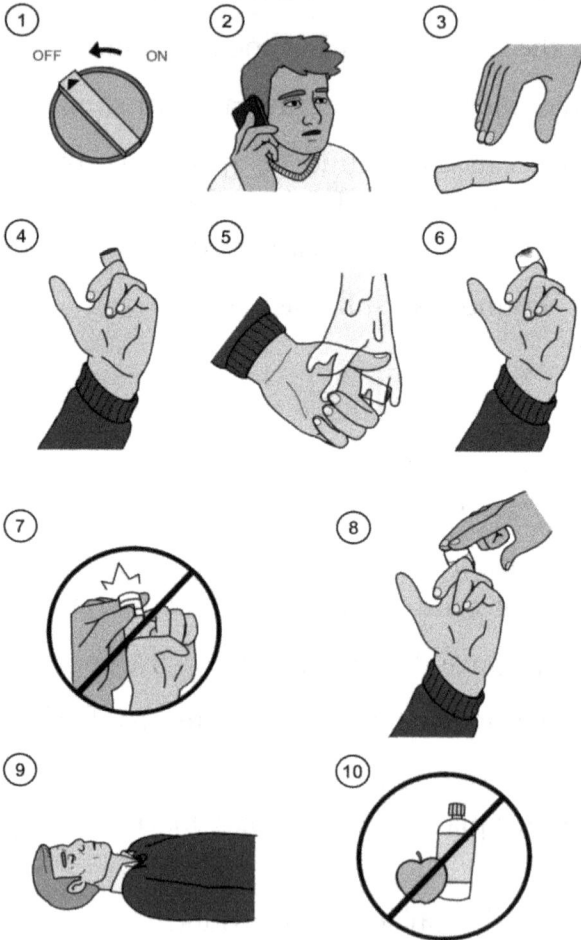

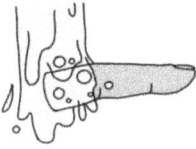

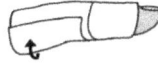

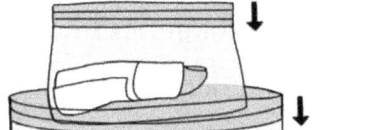

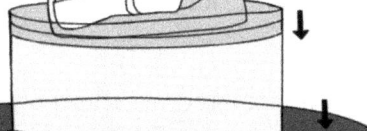

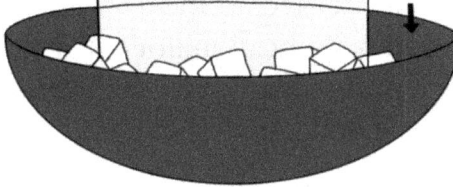

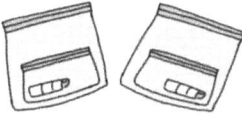

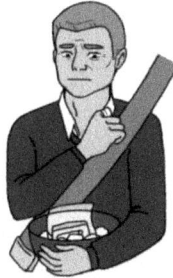

## Head Injuries

Most head injuries, from bumps to scrapes to cuts, are minor injuries that heal well with no professional medical care required. These minor injuries can be treated in the same way as we would bumps, scrapes, and cuts to other areas of the body. However, other head injuries can be life-threatening, from seemingly minor head bumps to concussions from contact sports.

## Common Causes of Head Injuries

- Car crashes are responsible for almost half of adult head injuries, with young adults and teenagers most likely to sustain head injuries in car crashes.
- Falls in children under 5-years-old, and in older adults above 60.
- Sports and work-related accidents. Men have double the chance of sustaining head injuries than women at work and during sports. Many sports-related head injuries may not be reported.
- Violent attacks and assaults often result in head injuries, with gunshot wounds accounting for the leading cause of death from a head injury.

## Signs of Head Injuries

- Severe facial or head bleeding
- Bleeding or fluid oozing from the ears and nose
- Vomiting
- Severe headache
- Change in consciousness that lasts more than a few seconds
- Black and blue discoloration below the eyes and behind the ears
- Not breathing
- Confusion

- Agitation
- Loss of balance
- Weakness or the inability to use limbs
- Unequal pupil size
- Slurred speech
- Blurred vision

In addition, children may also show these signs:

- Persistent crying
- Refusal to eat
- Bulging in the soft spot in front of the head in infants
- Repeated vomiting

## Treating Head Injuries

Your priority: Keep their head and neck still. Stop the bleeding and assist with breathing if necessary.

1. Keep the person's head still.

2. Get them to lie down and elevate their shoulders. Avoid moving the person's neck or relocating them unless absolutely necessary. If they are wearing headgear such as a helmet, don't remove it.

3. Stop bleeding by applying direct pressure with sterile gauze or cloth unless you suspect a skull fracture.

4. Monitor the person for changes in breathing and alertness. If you find no breathing, heartbeat, coughing or other movements, begin CPR.

5. If the person is stable, look for signs or injury to other parts of the body and attend to them if needed.

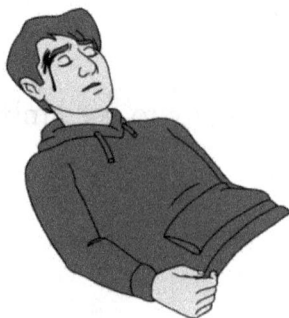

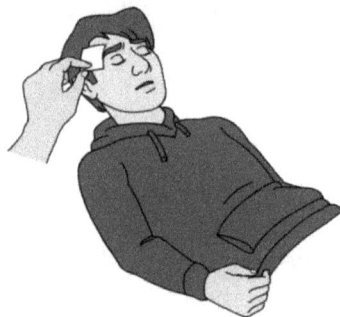

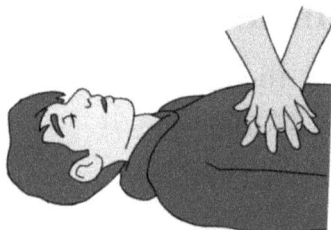

## Concussion

Concussion occurs when the brain comes into sharp contact with the inside of the skull from a blow to the head or a fall. Severe concussions can be dangerous if the person loses consciousness. It is vital to avoid sports and other activities that might result in a second concussion as a second impact can often lead to permanent brain damage or even be fatal if the first concussion is not fully healed. People may take between three months to a year to recover fully from a serious concussion.

## Signs and Symptoms of Concussion

- Stare blankly (be dazed)
- Appear confused or cry for no reason
- Nausea
- Vomiting
- Headache
- Dizziness
- Memory loss (including amnesia)
- Blurry vision
- Ringing in the ears (tinnitus)
- Loss of taste and smell
- Irritability
- Slurred speech
- Sensitivity to light and noise.

When mild symptoms persist, medical care must be found.

Sometimes a person may experience post concussive syndrome for three months or even a year after the injury. Symptoms include blurred vision, forgetfulness, concentration problems, nausea, headache, and vomiting. Sometimes, there may be a change in personality, problems with balance and a lack of coordination, disruption of sleep patterns, depression and other psychological disorders, fatigue, and bouts of dizziness.

# Assisting Someone Suffering from Concussion

Your priority: Monitor the person to determine if their symptoms are worsening and relay any information to medical professionals. If they have a severe concussion, it is best to wake them up gently every hour if medical help is delayed. If a child or infant shows signs of concussion, always get them swift medical care.

At home:

1. If you find the person's eyes are dilated (pupils are very large), they have difficulty walking and maintaining their balance, or they can't hold a conversation, then wake them up every couple of hours and get them urgent medical attention.

2. If the person doesn't show the symptoms from 1., then it is safe and good for them to get as much rest as they need.

3. Ensure the person avoids sports and other heavy, physically demanding activities as well as driving.

4. Manage mentally demanding activities so they have less stress and more rest.

5. Recommend less exposure to electronic screens, including phones and avoiding alcohol and non-prescription drugs.

# Poisoning

Poison is a toxic substance that makes a person feel sick or causes injuries to their mind and body. Over ninety percent of poisoning occurs at home. (Healthwise staff, 2018) Poisons are found in all households in the form of cleaning aids, houseplants, cosmetics, and even medication or supplements taken in the wrong dose or by someone who does not need the medication. Industrial chemicals are also toxic and can be found in homes and at work.

Poisons can cause harm when they are eaten, drunk, inhaled, in contact with your skin or your eyes. Products that give off fumes are generally considered poisonous, as are substances found in aerosol form.

## Signs and Symptoms of Poisoning

Symptoms of poisoning can often be mistaken for seizures, strokes, insulin reactions, alcohol intoxication and other conditions.

Look for these signs and symptoms:

- Burns and redness around mouth and lips
- Breath that smells of chemicals such as paint thinner or gasoline
- Vomiting
- Difficulty breathing
- Drowsiness
- Confusion or other altered mental state

## Treating Poisoning

Your priority: Identify the poison, remove contaminated clothing, assist in breathing, apply suitable steps to minimize harm from the identified poison. Use a facemask or pocket mask if you are to give CPR.

Note: Never induce vomiting in the person!

Stay calm and follow the steps below in order. Act as quickly as possible.

1. Check if the person is conscious.

2. Open the airway, ensuring their tongue isn't blocking their throat. Tilt their head back and lift their chin up with your forefinger and thumb while gently pressing their forehead back with your other hand. Position the person on their back. See Opening The Airway for more instructions.

3. Check if the person is breathing: look for the belly or chest moving up and down; feel the chest move up and down; feel the patient's breath on your cheek; put your ear close to the person's mouth and listen for sounds of their breathing.

4. If the person is not breathing after you've opened the airway, clear out the mouth and the throat. Turn their head to one side. Using one or two fingers, and preferably using gloves, scoop around the mouth and throat to clear out any vomit. Take care not to lodge any foreign objects down their throat. If the person wears false teeth, remove the dentures. If the person resumes breathing, turn them on their side into the recovery position. Check their pulse and breathing often. If the person doesn't resume breathing, you will need to help them breathe.

5. Give mouth-to-mouth respiration or mouth to nose respiration for an adult.

6. Check for a heartbeat. Feel for a pulse on the neck, in the hollow between the voice box and the muscle. Place two fingers on the Adam's Apple (voice box) and slide your fingers into the groove under the jaw. Feel for a pulse by holding your fingers in this position for at least five seconds. If the person has no pulse, they are in cardiac arrest. They will be unconscious, and their pupils will be large. Their skin will take on a blue-gray or ashen tinge or look for a blue tinge under their nails, to their lips, and the inside of their lower lids.

7. If they are in cardiac arrest, their breathing will also have stopped, and they will need both heart massage and mouth-to-mouth respiration. If their heart is beating, but they are not breathing, continue with mouth-to-mouth respiration. Take a deep breath and blow every five seconds until the person resumes breathing without help. You may need to do this for an hour. When the person starts to breathe, turn them onto their side and into the recovery position. The person may vomit when they resume breathing, but with them on their side, the vomit won't block their airway. Let the vomit drain out and then clear out their mouth with a finger.

8. If their heart is still not beating, give a heart massage.

How to Give a Heart Massage to an Adult

1. Check for a heartbeat. If there's none, commence with the heart massage.

2. On a firm surface, lay the person on their back. Kneel beside their chest.

3. Locate the right position to place your hands. From the lower edge of the ribs, follow the lower edge of the ribs to where they meet the breastbone. Place your middle finger at the base of the breastbone and your index finger next to it. Then place the heel of your other hand next to these two fingers, on the breastbone on the midline of the chest.

4. Cover your hand with your other hand and interlock your fingers so they are not touching the chest. Center your shoulders about the person's midline and straighten your arms.

5. Press down once on the lower half of the breastbone about four to five centimeters, keeping your arms straight. Then stop pressing. Count "And one and two and three" pressing down once for each count so you're doing 80 presses a minute. Presses must be regular and smooth, not jabs.

6. Remember to give mouth-to-mouth resuscitation after every 15 presses. Tilt the head back to open the airway, seal your mouth over the person's mouth and give two breaths.

7. Continue with the two breaths for every 15 presses. After one minute, check for a heartbeat, then again after three minutes,

then after every 12 cycles. As soon as the heartbeat resumes, stop the heart massage. The person's color may return to normal and their pupils may constrict.

8. Continue mouth-to-mouth respiration until the person breathes without help. It may take some time for breathing to resume even though the heart is now beating. When breathing resumes, position the person on their side in the recovery position. If you have another person to assist you, work as a team and get them to do the breathing while you do the heart massage.

9. If the person is unconscious, ensure they are in the recovery position.

10. Give first aid for fits (convulsions) if necessary.

11. Thoroughly wash any chemicals out of the person's eyes before washing the person's skin as any delay worsens the person's condition. Use lots of cool, clean water.

12. Gently brush or wipe off any powder, liquid, or residue from the person's face. Get the person to sit or lie down with their head tilted back and turned to the side worst affected. Open the person's affected eye (or eyes) and pour or run cold water over it, ensuring the water runs away from the person's body and doesn't cause any more harm. Though the person may be in great discomfort or pain, allowing them to keep their eyes closed will cause permanent

damage. Gently, continue washing out the person's eye or eyes for 15 or 20 minutes, using a watch or a timer to ensure it is a full 15 to 20 minutes.

13. Ensure the inner lids are well rinsed. Ensure you've removed all solid pieces and residue of the chemical from between the folds of the eyes, the eyelashes, the eyebrows, and the hollows of the eyes. If you are not sure you've removed all traces of the chemical, then continue flushing out the eye for another 10 minutes.

14. Prevent the person from rubbing their eyes.

15. The person must be examined by a doctor as damage may be delayed.

16. If the person's eyes are sensitive to light, cover the eye with a sterile eye pad or dry gauze pad. If no sterile pads are available, use a clean folded cloth.

17. Secure the pad with a bandage, but not too tightly, to help heal the eye.

18. Remove all contaminated clothing and wash the person's skin and hair.

a) Move the person to the nearest shower or suitable water source. If no water is available, gently wipe or dab the person's skin and hair with paper or cloth. Don't rub or scrub the person's skin.

b) Bathe the person's injury under cool or lukewarm running water, using a mild soap if available. If no running water is available, use buckets of water. Bathe the person as quickly as you can, using lots of water. Remember to protect yourself from the chemical. Use an apron and gloves if they are at hand. Avoid breathing in chemical fumes.

c) While bathing the person, remove any contaminated clothing, including that with vomit, and any shoes and wristwatches. It is important to work speedily. Cut out clothing contaminated by corrosive or highly poisonous substances.

d) If the person has multiple or large areas of contamination, wash them under a shower or use a hose. If necessary, remember to sluice their hair, in the groin, under their fingernails, and behind their ears. Continue to run water over the person for at least ten minutes. If you can still see chemicals on the person, or their skin feels soapy or sticky, continue washing them down until their skin feels normal. This may take up to an hour.

e) Ensure that all the water is draining away quickly and safely as it will be contaminated by the chemical.

f) Dry the person's skin gently with a clean, soft towel. If clothing remains stuck to their skin even after bathing them, don't attempt to remove the cloth.

g) As poisons can seep through skin quickly, look for signs of poisoning.

h) Put contaminated clothes in a separate sealed container. Wash thoroughly before use. Throw out shoes that are contaminated. If cloth and paper were used to wash the person, put them in a sealed container and burn them.

**13.** Give first aid for poisonous bites and stings.

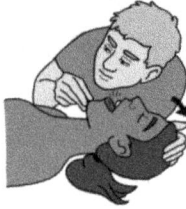

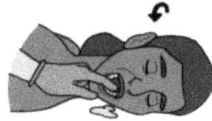

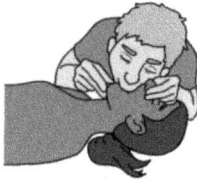

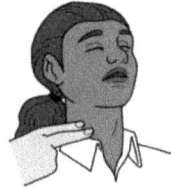

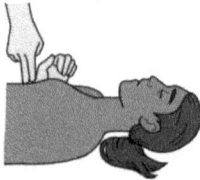

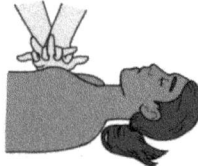

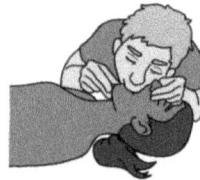

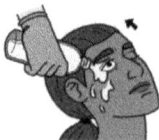

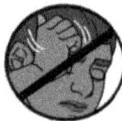

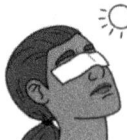

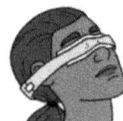

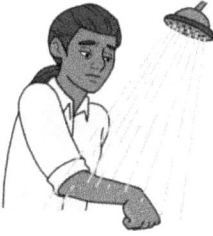

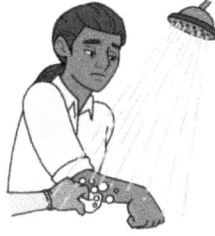

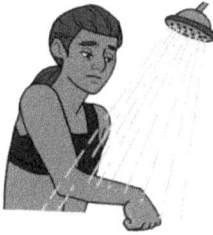

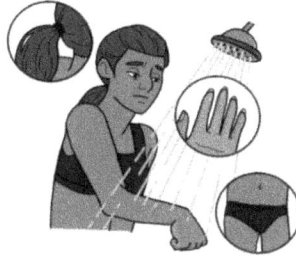

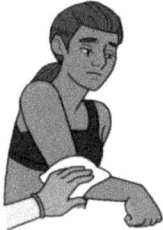

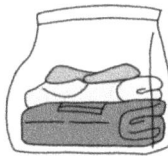

## Heat Stroke

When a person's body temperature rises quickly and they can't cool themselves sufficiently, heat stroke occurs. A person can easily be overcome by heat stroke without being aware of it by staying in a hot environment for too long or by undertaking strenuous activity in the heat. Heat stroke is dangerous as it causes damage to a person's brain and other vital organs. Children and animals (particularly those left in cars) are very susceptible to heat stroke, as are the elderly.

## Signs and Symptoms

- Fever of 104 F (40 C) or higher
- Changes in behavior such as slurred speech, agitation, or confusion
- Hot, dry skin or heavy sweating
- Nausea and vomiting
- Flushed skin
- Rapid pulse
- Rapid breathing
- Headache
- Fainting (usually the first sign in older adults)

## Treating Heat Stroke

Your priority: Move the person out of the heat and cool their bodies down as quickly as possible, then hydrate the person.

1. Quickly move the person out of the heat.
2. Remove restrictive and heavy clothing.
3. Cool them in the best way you can including:

a) Place the person under a cool shower or in a cool tub.

b) Spray with a garden hose.

c) Sponge with cold water.

d) Fan while misting with cold water.

e) Place ice packs, wet towels, or cold compresses under the armpits, groin and neck.

f) Cover with cool, damp sheets.

4. Feed the person cool water to rehydrate.

5. Don't allow the person sugary, caffeinated, or alcoholic drinks. Cold and icy beverages should also be avoided as they will cause stomach cramps.

6. Begin CPR if the person stops breathing and loses consciousness, showing no sign or circulation, coughing or other movements.

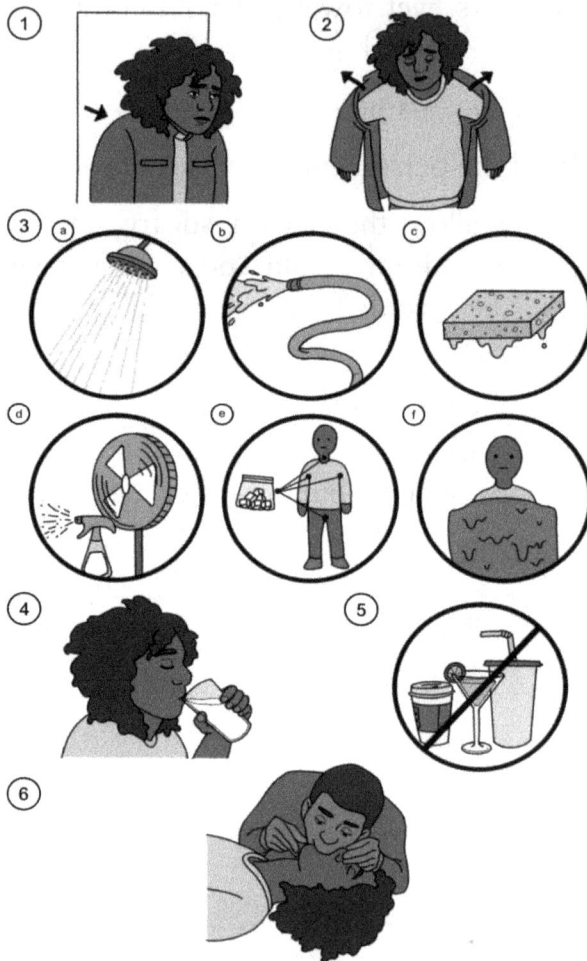

# Hypothermia and Frostbite

## Hypothermia

When your body loses heat faster than it can produce it, and your temperature drops below 95 F (35 C), you experience hypothermia. Untreated hypothermia quickly becomes life-threatening.

Hypothermia occurs when a person has prolonged exposure to cold in any season; from cold weather to immersion in cold water to exposure to indoor cooling below 50 F (10 C). The risk of hypothermia is increased by exhaustion and dehydration.

## Signs and Symptoms of Hypothermia

Symptoms of hypothermia develop gradually and may include:

- Shivering, which may stop as the condition worsens and the person's body temperature drops
- Slurred speech or mumbling
- Slow, shallow breathing
- Weakness
- Clumsiness of lack of coordination
- Drowsiness or low energy
- Confusion or memory loss
- Loss of consciousness
- Bright red, cold skin (in infants)

## What Not to Do in the Event of Hypothermia

- Don't rapidly warm the person up with a heating lamp or hot bath.
- Don't attempt to warm the arms and legs of the person as this may stress their heart.

- Don't give the person cigarettes or alcohol. Alcohol complicates the body's heating process and can exacerbate the situation. Cigarettes hinder circulation that is required to help the person recover.

## Treating Hypothermia

Your priority: Keep the person from further cold, raise their core temperature gradually without rubbing their limbs.

1. Move the person out of the cold as gently as possible.

2. If there is no shelter, shield the person from the wind, particularly their head and neck. Insulate them from the cold ground.

3. Gently remove wet clothing. Replace with dry, warm coats and blankets.

4. If more warmth is required, apply it gradually. For example, help heat the person's core by applying hot compresses to the torso of the body—neck, chest and groin. The CDC recommends using an electric blanket, if available. If you are using heat packs or hot water bottles, wrap them in towels first.

5. Feed the person warm, sweet, non-alcoholic drinks.

6. Begin CPR if the person slips into unconsciousness and shows no signs of life—no sign of breathing, coughing or movement.

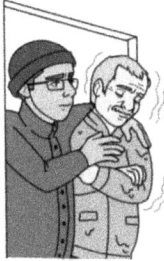 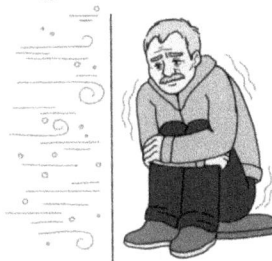

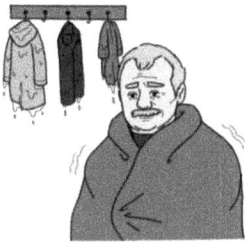 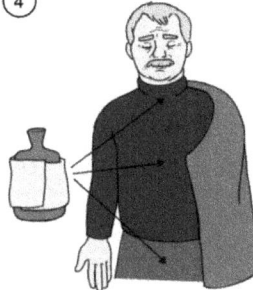

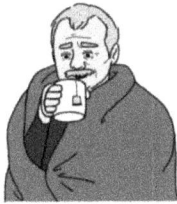 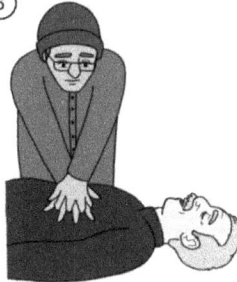

## Frostbites Vs Hypothermia

Frostbite occurs when your skin freezes during exposure to cold weather or water. It is common and often underestimated during winter fun activities but can still cause damage to your body.

While hypothermia is more serious and affects your body as a whole, frostbite, though localized, damages skin cells and tissue in the exposed parts of your skin by freezing them. Children, the elderly, people with hypertension or diabetes, smokers, alcohol consumers, and drug users are most at risk from frostbite.

Symptoms of frostbite include feelings of "pins and needles," numbness, swelling, blisters, loss of coordination and blackened skin.

While frostbite might seem less severe than hypothermia, the long-term effects of untreated and repeated frostbite are costly. Nerves may be damaged, affecting your sensitivity, while frostbite arthritis may affect you years later. Frostbite arthritis causes swelling and stiffness of your joints.

## Prevention of Frostbite

Dress according to the weather with layers and windproof and waterproof gear. Ensure your fingers and toes are protected. Avoid recreational drugs, alcohol, and heavy exercise when in icy winds. Ensure you are hydrating. Go out in the cold only if necessary and keep trips short. Ensure your clothing and shoes don't cut off your circulation.

## Treating Frostbite

Your priority: Remove wet clothing, gently warm skin with warm water.

Self-treatment:

1. Prioritize staying warm and preventing freezing again to avoid further skin damage.

2. To warm up:

a. Remove any wet clothing.

b. Elevate the frostbitten area slightly. Don't rub frostbitten areas as this can cause tissue damage.

c. Warm your skin by soaking in warm water that is about 105 F (40.5 C). Don't use heat sources to warm your skin such as heaters, fires, or electric blankets.

d. Be careful not to burn the area with hot water as the skin will be numb and burning the area will cause more damage to your skin. Once your fingers are soft again, remove them from the warm water.

e. Cover the frostbitten area with a sterile (clean) cloth. If your fingers or toes were affected, ensure they are wrapped individually to avoid stress and pressure on them.

f. Try to keep the area affected immobile. Don't walk with frostbitten feet.

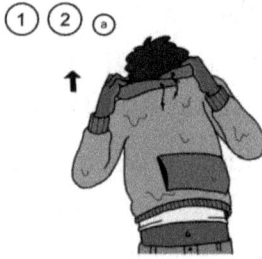

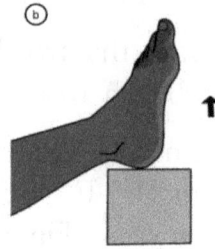

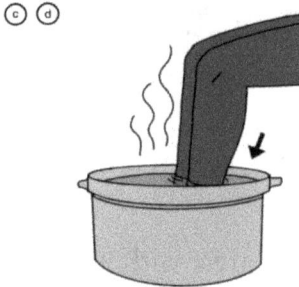

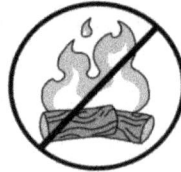

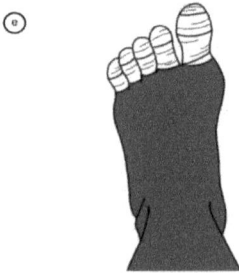

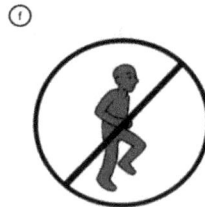

## Fractures

Bones are often fractured in accidents and falls. When there's no wound on the skin, it's a simple fracture.

## General Symptoms and Signs of Fracture

- Pain at or near the point of the fracture

- Discomfort and tenderness when pressure is applied over the area of the fracture

- Swelling in the affected area may make it difficult to identify or assess the extent of the fracture. Take care to detect other signs of fracture.

- Deformity of the limb

- Irregularity of the bone

## Treating Fractures

Your priority: Stop the bleeding if there is any and immobilize the limb with a splint.

1. Treat the fracture immediately. Unless in a life-threatening environment, don't move the person until the fractured limb has been immobilized. If necessary, immobilize the limb temporarily, then move the person as short a distance as possible to a safer area where a sturdier fix can be done.

2. Bleeding and open wounds must be attended to first, before the setting of the fracture.

3. Steady and support the injured area first, ensuring the person cannot bend or move the limb. This prevents further injury and bleeding, as well as minimizes the risk of broken splinters of bone causing internal injury to muscle, skin, nerves, and blood vessels.

4. Splint the limb with bandages or other suitable items so the limb is completely immobilized.

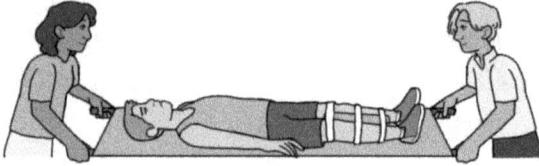

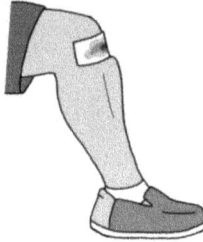

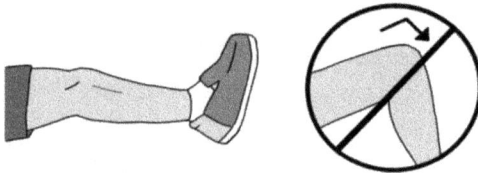

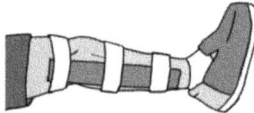

## Electrocution

When a person touches a live or naked wire, cable or rail, the shock experienced can range from mild to severe. In the case of severe shock, a burn will result. In the case of high voltages, burns may be severe or deep.

A live current passing through a person's body can be life-threatening and result in cardiac arrest and other injuries.

Any electrocution can be fatal; a high voltage is not necessary.

When a shock has occurred, swift action can save a person's life.

## Treating Electrocution

If the person is still in contact with the electric current, do not touch them.

Your priority: Remove the source of the current from the person and, if it's safe for you to do so, assist the person with breathing and circulation.

1. Switch off the current or cut off the supply by unplugging the source of the shock, wrenching it free or breaking the cable, taking care not to touch the live end yourself. If that's not possible, move the source away from you and the person with a non-conductive, dry object made from cardboard, plastic, or wood. Never use metal or attempt to cut a cable with a knife or scissors.

2. With utmost care, remove the person from contact with the current using dry, insulated materials. At home, use a folded garment, gloves, or newspaper for protection.

3. Reassure the patient.

4. Lay the person on their back with their head positioned so that it is low and turned to one side unless they are injured on their head, chest or abdomen; then raise their head and shoulders slightly and ensure their head is supported.

5. Loosen clothing around their neck, chest, and waist.

6. Do not give the person any fluids until the paramedics arrive.

7. Begin CPR if the person isn't breathing, has no heartbeat, or otherwise shows no signs of circulation.

8. Keep the person from getting chilled.

9. Apply a sterile gauze bandage or a clean cloth to any burn areas. Never use a towel or a blanket as the loose fibers can stick to the burns.

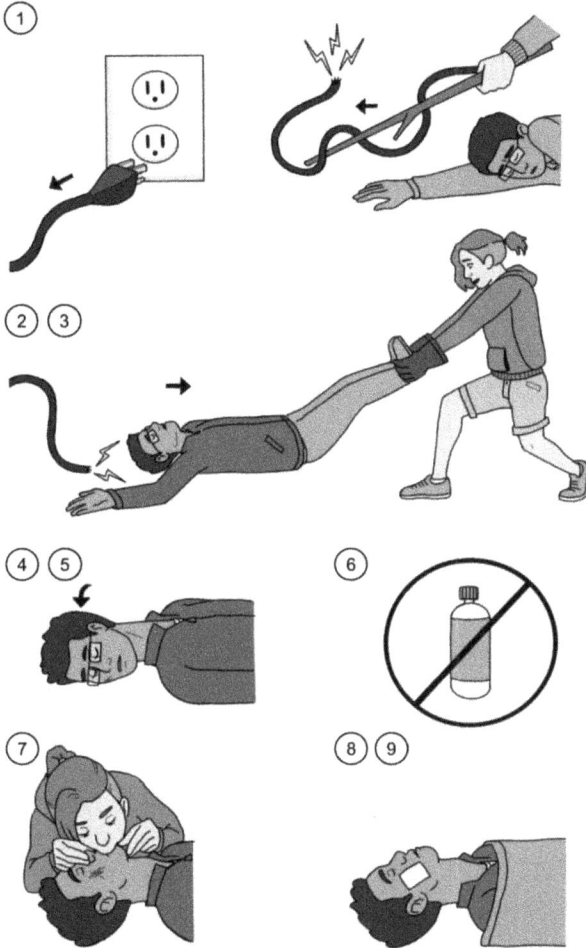

# Clothes on Fire

Fire is a common urgency that is horrifying in its ability to cause us to panic and escalate into a disaster. If a person's clothes catch fire, use the Stop, Drop, Roll method then ensure the fire is under control.

# Helping Someone with Their Clothes on Fire

Your priority: Roll the person (if they have no neck, head, or spinal injury) on the floor to snuff out the fire.

1.  Stop. Reassure the person and talk to them calmly through the next two steps. If they are panicking, be firm and do the actions with them.

2.  Drop. Drop to the ground as swiftly as possible. Cover them with a non-flammable coat, rug, or fire blanket if possible.

3.  Roll immediately. Help the person roll their body. This should snuff out the fire on their clothes.

4.  Assess any burns.

5.  Call emergency services.

6.  Treat any burns until help arrives.

# Difficulty in Swimming or Drowning

Children, pets, and the elderly can often fall into water or experience difficulty while swimming in water.

Your priority: Help them out of the water only if it is safe for you to do so. Prevent water from damaging lungs and brain. Assist in breathing if necessary and keep them warm. Get the person to a medical facility to prevent secondary drowning—when air passages swell hours after lungs are affected by immersion in water.

# Helping Someone Immersed in Water or Drowning

1. Don't get into the water if you are not a trained lifesaver. Dial emergency services or call for help.

2. If it is safe to do so, hold out a hand, a stick, or throw a floating object.

3. Assist the person out of the water, ensuring you don't fall in yourself.

4. Keep them warm.

5. Set them in the recovery position, preferably with their head lower than the rest of their body so they can't inhale any more water.

6. Ensure their airways are clear.

7. Remove wet clothing if dry clothes are available and treat them for hypothermia.

8. Arrange for transport to a medical facility with a doctor.

# Caring for Someone in Isolation or Quarantine at Home

Only one adult should care for the person or come into any contact with them. If this adult is you, ensure that should you be sick, another elected able adult or the oldest teenager can take over your duties and knows whom to contact for help. Ensure the stand-by carer is not pregnant.

Your priority: Tend to the isolating person's daily needs with food, water, medication and any other help they may require. Avoid the infection yourself. Monitor the person for aggravated symptoms of the infection.

## Points to Remember

- Keep the isolating person away from others in the home. The isolating person should stay in a bedroom with the door closed, and preferably, if possible, have a bathroom for their own use only.

- Don't allow any visitors.

- Keep pets away from the isolating person as pets can become infected by certain diseases, too. Also, it is harder and more traumatic to disinfect pets regularly than it is for people.

- Keep all items used by the isolating person separate from those of the general household. This includes bedding and linen, toiletries, cutlery, mugs, dinnerware, and unwashed clothes. Handle the isolating person's laundry with gloves or plastic bags on your hands.

- Ensure the isolating person rests and is well nourished.

- Encourage the isolating person to exercise if they are well enough to do so.

- When interacting with other people, for example in the garden or other common areas, wear a well-fitted mask and stay at least 1.5 meters (5 ft) away.

- Always disinfect the area the isolating person has been in with a reputable disinfectant.

- Wash your hands often.

- Monitor the isolating person for any further symptoms or deterioration of their condition. If they do produce symptoms or their condition worsens, get medical help.

- If you have applied first aid to an isolating person, take extra precautions with wound treatment and CPR, and ensure all waste is specially marked and incinerated at a suitable facility.

- If you've called for medical help for a person in isolation, let the dispatchers know that the person in distress is isolating.

As for the rest of the household:

- Maintain a positive attitude.

- Discuss the infection openly and ensure everyone is informed about the health of the person in quarantine.

- Keep the household routine as normal as possible.

- Exercise regularly, outdoors if possible, to alleviate stress and depression.

- Maintain contact with family and friends via conference calling or messaging.

- Remember quarantines usually end after a two-week period and that you and your family have the resilience to cope.

## Chapter 5
# Responding to Emergencies Related to Permanent Medical Conditions

A person with a permanent medical condition can sometimes find themselves in an emergency medical situation resulting from their chronic illness. We will look at how to deal with some of the more common emergencies resulting from chronic health conditions such as epileptic seizures, heart attacks, and severe allergic reactions.

## Heart Attacks and Chest Pains

Heart attacks occur when the flow of blood to the heart is blocked. Blockages may be caused by blood clots, blood plaque (cholesterol) in arteries, or collapsed blood vessels. Treatment during the first 90 minutes of an attack greatly increases the chance the person's life will be saved.

While not all chest pains are a sign of heart attack, it usually denotes a medical condition and you should ensure that the person gets medical attention.

## Symptoms for Both Genders

- Discomfort and pain in the chest area; or a feeling of pressure, tightness, or an aching and squeezing sensation at the center of the chest for more than 15 minutes.

- Pain that spreads to the shoulders, arms, neck, back, jaw, teeth, and sometimes the abdomen.

- Indigestion, heartburn, nausea, vomiting, or abdominal pain

- Shortness of breath

- Dizziness, fainting, light-headedness

- Sweating

- A racing or irregular heartbeat

**Specific Symptoms for Men**

Most men experience cold sweats while pain may travel down their left arm.

**Specific Symptoms for Women**

Women tend to have more indistinct symptoms such as nausea, stomach upsets, dizziness, tiredness, shortness of breath, jaw, or back pain.

# Treating Heart Attacks

1. If the medication is available, give the person an aspirin, or if they have a doctor's prescription for nitroglycerin, then ensure they take the correct dosage at once. Aspirin reduces the incidences of blood clots and reduces damage to the heart if the person is experiencing a heart attack.

2. If you don't have access to medication and the person is unconscious, is not breathing and you find no pulse, begin CPR. Press hard and fast in a rapid rhythm of 100 to 120 presses a minute.

# Stroke

When a blood vessel in the brain bursts or is blocked, a person has a stroke. With its oxygen and blood cut off, the affected part of the brain begins to die, and the body functions that part of the brain controls are not available to the person. For instance, they may not be able to speak if their speech centers are affected.

It is important to know the signs of stroke and to act fast as brain damage can occur within minutes of the stroke. Receiving medical help quickly not only reduces brain damage, but also makes a full recovery possible.

## Signs of a Stroke

- Sudden weakness, numbness, tingling or loss of movement in the face, arm, or leg, particularly on one side of the body.
- Sudden vision loss in one eye: blurred vision, dim vision, or no vision
- Sudden speech problems
- Sudden confusion and no understanding of even simple statements
- Sudden problems with movement or balance; loss of bowel and bladder control
- Sudden severe headache unlike those usually experienced
- Quite often, most strokes are painless.

FAST is a simple way to remember the symptoms of stroke:

- F - face drooping

- A - arm weakness
- S - Speech difficulty
- T - Time to call 911

## Treating Stroke Victims

1. Ensure they are in a safe, comfortable position and environment. Lay them on their side with their head supported in case they vomit.

2. Check their breathing. If they stop breathing, administer CPR. If they're having trouble breathing, loosen tight clothing such as ties and scarves.

3. Reassure them by talking to them in a calm tone.

4. Keep them warm. Cover them with a blanket.

5. If they are weak, particularly in a limb, don't move them.

6. Observe the person for a change in their condition. Be prepared to tell emergency operators and responders the person's symptoms and when they first appeared. If the person fell and hit their head, mention that as soon as possible.

7. Perform CPR as needed.

8. Stay calm and alert.

## What Not to Do in the Case of Stroke

- Don't allow the person any drink or food.

- Don't drive to the hospital. Wait for emergency services.

- Don't give the person any medication.

- The key to stroke treatment is getting hospital treatment as soon as possible. Patients taken to hospital in an ambulance get diagnosed and are treated much quicker than a patient not arriving in an ambulance.

## Seizures

Seizures may be caused by epilepsy, as a reaction to incorrect medication, or other medical or traumatic reasons.

### Signs and Symptoms

- Loss of consciousness

- Muscle contractions and convulsions

- Weakness

- Clouded awareness

- Loss of sensation

- Fidgeting

- Strange sensations in the stomach

- Confusion and sleepiness after the seizure

### In the Event of a Seizure

Your aim is to keep the person safe until the seizure stops.

1. Loosen any clothing around the person's neck.

2. Lay them on the floor.

3. Don't attempt to restrain them or put any objects in their mouth.

4. Clear the area and ensure there are no hard objects nearby.

5. Stay with them until the seizure stops.

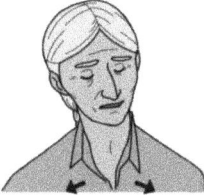

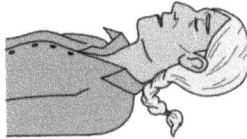

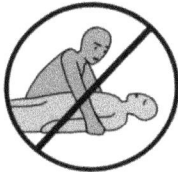

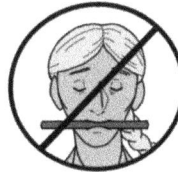

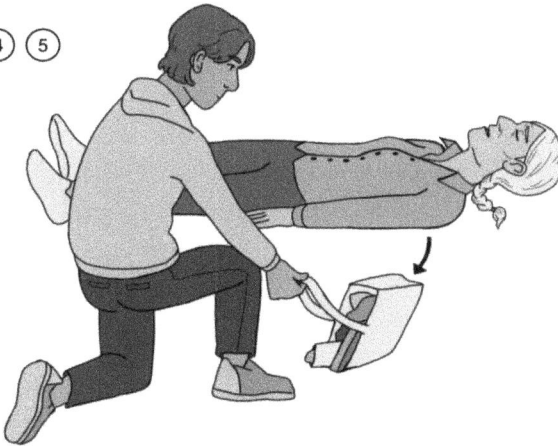

# Severe Allergic Reactions or Anaphylaxis

A severe allergic reaction (anaphylaxis) can be life-threatening as it may cause a shock, a sudden drop in blood pressure, or interfere with breathing.

People with allergies may experience reactions minutes after exposure to the allergen. Sometimes there can be a delay before anaphylaxis occurs, or even no apparent trigger.

## Signs and Symptoms

- Skin reactions including rashes, paleness, red skin, itching or hives
- Swelling on the face, lips, eyes, or throat.
- Constriction of the throat with wheezing or trouble breathing
- A weak and rapid pulse
- Diarrhea, nausea, vomiting
- Dizziness, fainting or losing consciousness.

Treating a Person with a Severe Allergic Reaction

Your aim is to help the person use their allergy medication, assist them with breathing if necessary, and get them to a medical care facility.

1. Ask the person if they are carrying an epinephrine auto injector (Epipen, Auvi-Q,or others) to treat an allergy attack.

2. If the person has an auto injector, ask them whether you should help them inject the

medication. This is usually done by pressing the auto injector against the person's thigh.

3. Lay the person down on their back. Keep them still.

4. Loosen tight clothing and cover the person with a blanket. Don't give them anything to drink.

5. If they are vomiting or bleeding from the mouth, turn them to their side so the fluids can drain and they won't choke.

6. If the person stops breathing and shows no signs of coughing or other movement, begin CPR. Do uninterrupted compressions of about 100 every minute until paramedics arrive.

7. Get the person emergency medical treatment. After anaphylaxis, monitoring at a hospital is usually necessary as symptoms can reoccur.

## What Not to Do

- Don't delay treatment by waiting to see if symptoms improve. Seek immediate emergency treatment. In severe cases, death can result within half an hour.

- An antihistamine pill isn't a sufficient treatment for anaphylaxis. While they may relieve symptoms, they can't fight off the damage a severe allergic reaction does to the body.

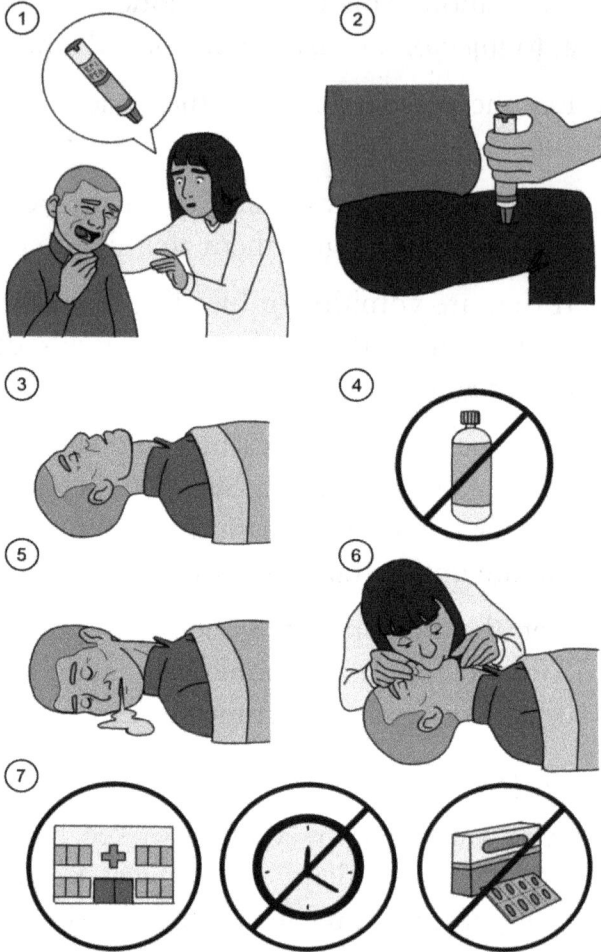

## Asthma

Asthma is so prevalent that every ten seconds someone in the world is having a potentially life-threatening attack. (NHS Choices. 2019) Their chances of having a severe attack is greatly reduced if they are on the right treatment.

## Signs and Symptoms

Take action when the following signs and symptoms worsen:

- Coughing, wheezing, tightness in their chest, or breathlessness

- Their usual reliever or inhaler isn't helping

- Feeling too breathless to talk, eat, or sleep

- Breathing rate is going up and they still cannot catch their breath

- The person's peak flow score is lower than normal

- Children, in addition, may complain of chest or stomach ache.

## Treating an Asthma Attack

1. Sit the person upright (not lying down), and coach them to take slow, steady breaths.

2. Reassure them and help them remain calm as panicking will worsen their condition.

3. Encourage them to take long, deep breaths. This helps to prevent hyperventilation by slowing down their breathing. Have them breathe in through their nose and out through their mouth.

4. Help them move away from the trigger and into clean air or an air-conditioned place. The asthma attack could be triggered by dust, cigarette smoke, or the smell of chemicals such as ammonia, chlorine gas or sulfur dioxide.

5. Give them a hot caffeinated beverage. This may help open their airways a little and provide relief for a short while.

6. Let them take one puff of their usual inhaler every 30 to 60 seconds for a maximum of 10 puffs.

7. Repeat every 15 minutes.

8. If their condition improves, they don't require emergency medical care, but they do need to consult their doctor as soon as possible.

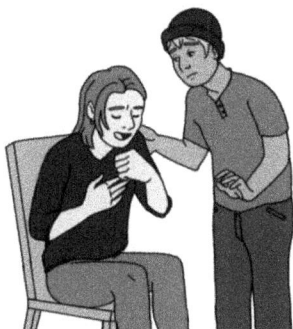
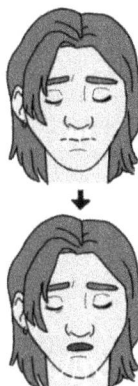

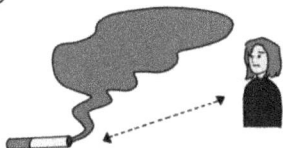

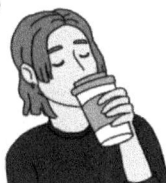
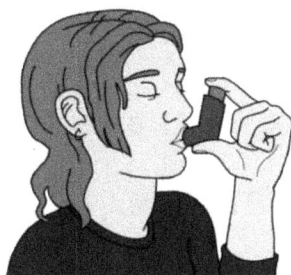

## Tachycardia or Heart Palpitations

Heart palpitations occur when the person feels as if their heart is pounding, or fluttering, at an alarmingly high rate. These palpitations may last for a few seconds and may occur at any time.

While not all palpitations are caused by a heart condition, they can be caused by other factors that put stress on your heart, such as illness, dehydration, general stress, exercise, caffeine, pregnancy, illegal drugs, or tobacco products.

## Treating Heart Palpitations

In most cases, no treatment is needed. You can help alleviate the person's condition by:

1. Trying relaxation techniques.
2. Giving them water to drink water.
3. Encouraging them to do vagal maneuvers.
4. Encouraging them to avoid stimulants.
5. Restoring electrolyte balance.

## Hyperglycemia

One of the two conditions resulting from diabetes, hyperglycemia occurs in any age group when a person with Type 1 diabetes runs out of insulin. As their bodies don't produce insulin, they are dependent on their insulin injections, pumps, and injection pen.

Hyperglycemia develops slowly over a few hours or days and often leads to a diabetic coma which must be treated in the hospital.

## Signs of Hyperglycemia

- Sweet breath with a fruity smell
- Hyperventilation or rapid breathing and pulse
- Drowsiness
- Warm, dry skin.

While you can't treat a diabetic coma and hyperglycemia, your priority is to call for immediate medical care and to monitor the person. If they lose consciousness and stop breathing, give them CPR until medical help arrives.

## Hypoglycemia

The second condition resulting from diabetes known as Type 2 hypoglycemia usually occurs in mature people or those suffering from obesity. As their body's sugar and insulin shifts out of balance, they become distressed and more ill.

Hyperglycemia develops fast if a meal is skipped or the person has exerted themselves too much. This condition often occurs in recently diagnosed diabetics who are still adjusting to their insulin regime and new lifestyle.

## Signs of Hypoglycemia

- Weakness, faintness, or hunger.
- Muscle tremors
- Weak pulse
- Palpitations
- Cold clammy skin
- Sweating
- Confusion, irritability, or irrationality
- The person may be aware of their condition and history of diabetes and carry medication or wear a bracelet
- Responses grow erratic

# Treating Hypoglycemia

Your priority: Raising the blood-sugar level of the person as fast as possible, then finding medical care.

1. Sit the person down as soon as possible.

2. If the person is carrying sugar, glucose, or candy, help them ingest them. If the person has no sugar products on them, give them two teaspoons of sugar, a hard sugar candy, or a cup of regular soda (not the diet variants), or fruit juice.

3. If the person is recovering well, feed them more food and drink and allow them to rest.

4. Once they're feeling much better, help them do their glucose test if they carry a personal kit, or to find medical help.

5. Monitor the person.

6. If the person doesn't respond well to sugar intake, look for other conditions for their distress and stay with them until professional medical care arrives.

# Chapter 6
# Alternative Medicine for Emergencies

You may not always have your medical kit at hand, but you may have your larder or other resources available that may help in an emergency. Alternative and herbal remedies have been used in emergency situations for centuries. We'll look at some of the alternative herbal remedies the Red Cross of America and others recommend for your first aid kit.

## Disclaimer

Natural remedies are extremely potent, interact with medications in unpredictable ways, and can be toxic and lead to poisoning or exacerbation of symptoms. If a person is allergic to any ingredient of a natural remedy, do not give it to them. Therefore, all homemade natural remedies must be precisely labeled with the ingredients (including carrier oils, alcohols, or other carrier and preserving agents), the date made, the expected expiration date, and dosage or instructions for use. These labels must be in indelible or waterproof ink.

Herbal remedies should be administered with great care or not at all (depending on the herb) to pregnant women, infants, young children, diabetics, people with high blood pressure, and people with existing kidney or liver conditions.

Herbs and spice-based remedies build up concentrations in your body the more often you take them. If taken over extended periods of time, this can lead to toxicity and illness. Therefore, herbal remedies should be taken in small doses (some even minuscule), and immune boosters and other supplements and preventative remedies should be taken on an on-and-off basis to allow concentrations to deplete safely.

If a person experiences an allergic reaction to an initial dose or other negative reaction, the preparation should no longer be used to treat them.

If you have been using herbal supplements to treat someone, inform any medical professional who takes over attending the ill or distressed person.

## Notes for Storing Natural Remedies in First Aid Kits

- Store ingredients in airtight containers.
- Wrap glass bottles in paper or cloth to prevent leakage and cushion them. Label on the outside.
- Ensure all ingredients, instructions for use, and dates are noted on the containers.
- Check powders regularly to ensure they are moisture-free.
- If an ointment, salve, cream smells 'off' or rancid, don't use it.

## Manuka Honey

Manuka honey usually doesn't spoil and can be kept safely in your first aid kit for long periods of time.

Use Manuka Honey for:

- Burns. Manuka honey is now widely accepted as an excellent treatment for burns and wounds. Even conventional medical care is using manuka honey in burn treatment as it has natural antiseptic properties and prevents bacteria and viruses from entering wounds.

- Sore throats. Slowly suck a teaspoon to relieve a sore throat.

- Energy boost. Eat the honey for a quick energy boost or for much-needed calories.

## Manuka Oil

Manuka oil has been shown to kill viruses (antiviral), bacteria (antibacterial), and fungi (antifungal).

Use Manuka Oil for:

- Skin abrasions
- Abscesses, blisters, bedsores, boils, sores
- Tonsillitis, ulcers, varicose veins
- Cold sores, acne, carbuncles, pimples
- Cracked skin, dermatitis, eczema
- Dandruff, fungal infections, lice, ringworm
- Infections from body piercings, insect bites, nail infections
- Rhinitis, sunburn, oily skin, tinea

## Colloidal Silver

Colloidal Silver is similar to Manuka in that it is used to prevent infections in wounds. It may treat food poisoning when taken in safe doses internally. It may also help manage eye infections with a few drops in the eye before bed. It has been known to also help with ear infections and to help alleviate stomach bugs. However, Colloidal Silver must be taken in the correct dosage if used internally as it may have side effects depending on the distillation.

## Live Aloe Vera

Clear sap from an aloe plant has similar wound healing and antibacterial uses as Manuka. As a broken leaf of the plant seals itself, you can carry the leaf with you.

Use Live Aloe Vera to:

- Apply directly to burns, cuts, and scrapes.
- Alleviate sunburn.
- Pack it in a flesh wound until medical help arrives.

Taken internally, aloe vera is believed to help relieve intestinal issues.

## Cayenne Pepper

Taken internally, cayenne pepper acts as a vasodilator, opening up blood vessels. It can be used for emergency stroke treatment, heart attacks, and is often used in conjunction with other herbs to deliver the properties of the other herbs via the bloodstream to the area needing treatment.

It is also believed to aid sluggish circulation by applying it to the skin or soaking feet in warm water with some cayenne pepper in it.

Cayenne pepper also works well as a muscle relaxant, either taken internally, or if applied topically with a cream.

# Black or Green Tea Bags

Black and green tea bags, or any caffeinated tea bag with large amounts of tannin, can be used to help stop bleeding. Wrap the wet tea bag in gauze and bite down on it to stop dental bleeding, or hold it against the wound, or secure it with a bandage on limbs and other areas of the body. (McDermott & Sullivan, 2017).

Green tea bags can also be used as a compress on eyes for conjunctivitis (place it on the eye for about 15 to 20 minutes), with the green tea being used as an eyewash. Green tea bags can also be used as a cold compress on skin irritations.

# Chamomile

Chamomile is anti-inflammatory and relaxes the body. Chamomile tea or salves can work as muscle relaxants and provide relief from skin irritation, sore muscles, and anxiety. Inhaling steam from an infusion of chamomile flowers or tea also helps provide relief from sinus congestion. Take care not to burn your skin with the steam.

# Arnica Gel or Cream

Arnica flowers improve circulation and have antibacterial properties.

To Use Arnica Gel or Cream:

- Apply it to sprain, strains, sore muscles.

- Apply it to bumps and bruises to reduce swelling.

- Taken internally as a liquid or homeopathic preparation, it can help relieve headaches and help tissues heal after surgery.

## Calendula Cream

Calendula cream is made from *Calendula Officinalis*, also known as marigolds. Use it to treat scrapes, cuts, bruises, and open sores. It can be used if no antibacterial or antiseptic wash is available.

## Rescue Remedy

Made from five Bach flower remedies, Rescue Remedy helps *you* stay calm when dealing with emergencies. Use it when dealing with physical shock and to keep you focused on following the steps to help a person in distress.

## Rubbing Alcohol and Hydrogen Peroxide

Both Rubbing Alcohol and Hydrogen Peroxide have very long shelf-lives and are very affordable.

Use Rubbing Alcohol and Hydrogen Peroxide to:

- Clean light wounds when water and soap aren't available.

- Treat colds and flu by dropping a 3% solution of hydrogen peroxide into the ear. However, if the person has an ear infection or a perforated eardrum, this is not recommended.

## Ginger

Ginger has long been used in the East for its strong anti-inflammatory, antimicrobial and digestive properties. Use a piece of fresh ginger about the size of your fingernail. Alternatively, allow the person to drink up to two cups of ginger a day as larger quantities of ginger can cause stomach irritation.

Use Ginger to:

- Settle an upset stomach
- Aid with digestion
- Relieve abdominal gas and cramping
- Treat bacteria-induced diarrhea
- Alleviate symptoms of food poisoning
- Fight viral infections such as colds and relieve some of the symptoms
- Help dissolve mucus congestion and to induce sweating to overcome a cold fever, or flu
- Relieve nausea and vomiting
- Relieve motion sickness
- Relieve morning sickness. However, great caution must be used as ginger in larger amounts can affect pregnancy
- Relieve a sore throat, coughing, post-nasal drip, and mucus congestion as it is a natural analgesic
- Relieve the pain and swelling from rheumatoid arthritis, gout, and osteoarthritis
- Relieve menstrual pain and cramps. Caution must be used as ginger may promote bleeding
- Provide relief from migraine pain, nausea, and dizziness as it can act as a pain blocker and reduce inflammation
- Lower cholesterol levels, blood pressure, and prevent blood clots so the risk of heart disease is reduced

- Fight allergic reaction, reduce asthma attacks, fight inflammation of the airways and fight respiratory viruses

## Activated Charcoal or Bentonite Clay

Activated charcoal and bentonite clay both work to reduce toxins and poisons, so are helpful in overcoming food poisoning and stomach upsets.

Mix it into a paste and apply it to insect bites and stings to remove the toxins.

Activated charcoal can also be used to filter water in remote locations if water of drinking quality is scarce or unavailable.

## Echinacea and Elderberry

Echinacea and elderberry are immune-boosting herbs that may shorten the duration of colds and the flu. Take at the first hint of exposure.

## Eucalyptus

Eucalyptus oil is a natural antibiotic and antiviral. Mix a few drops of the essential oil in a carrier oil such as olive oil or coconut oil and use a vapor rub.

Use eucalyptus to:

- Help open congested airways
- Treat colds
- Treat sinus problems
- Support treatment of respiratory problems

## Lavender

Lavender essential oil is often used to soothe and calm. Mix in a carrier oil before use.

Use Lavender to:

- Relieve headaches by rubbing onto the temples
- Reduce anxiety
- Treat insomnia
- Apply over the chest or over the feet for soothing relief

## Tea Tree Oil

Tea Tree oil is a natural antiseptic.

Use Tea Tree Oil to:

- Treat bacterial infections as an alternative to antibacterial cream
- Prevent infections
- Heal cuts and bruises
- Treat minor skin burns
- Repel fungal problems such as athlete's foot and infected toenails.
- Relieve discomfort from insect bites

## Witch Hazel

Witch Hazel is an astringent, antiseptic, and anti-inflammatory and is often used as a skin tonic and deodorant.

Use Witch Hazel to:

- Treat skin irritations such as rashes and insect bites
- Mix or dilute essential oils by using it as a carrier base

## Acupuncture and Acupressure

Acupuncture is the application of pressure or needles to special points in the body. It has been proven as an effective means of pain relief and is used extensively in the UK and Germany in conventional medical centers as part of pain management treatments.

NB! If you are not trained in acupressure, acupuncture, or massage, don't press too hard on these points. If the person experiences a high level of discomfort or is further distressed by acupressure, then switch to another treatment.

Don't use acupressure or acupuncture on a pregnant woman as this can induce contractions.

## Treatments with Acupuncture and Acupressure

To apply acupuncture to a point in the body, press down with one or two fingers at the point for about a minute. The correct point to treat will feel harder or be sore to the person being treated.

- For headaches: Between the thumb and forefinger, pinch the web of flesh.
- For nausea: Place three fingers on the wrist. At the point of the forearm next to the third finger, depress the crease or slight hollow just off-center for about a minute.

- For neck pain and migraines: Press the hollows at the back of the base of your skull.

- For heartburn and indigestion: Measure six finger widths from your navel and two below the end of your rib cage. Depress the middle of your torso at that point.

- For nosebleeds: Wrap twine, a ribbon, or a shoelace around the width of the palm. Ask the person to make a fist with that palm for about a minute to activate all the pressure points.

## Artemisia Annua

In combination with other medical preparations, this Chinese herb is now considered among the most effective treatments for malaria. Used in China since the 3rd century, the herb is now available in a tablet form for oral use.

## Recipes for First Aid Material

Sometimes, you may run out of salves, creams, and ointments to treat minor emergencies, burns, and stings and running to the pharmacy is not an option. Fortunately, you can make your own salves, creams, and ointments at home with a few ingredients. Remember to label your DIY first aid essentials with instructions and expiration date.

Next, you'll find some basic recipes to create a base for your cream, ointment, or salve. Variations will follow to help you create your own must-have soothing and antiseptic applications.

NB! Before using any of your own herbal creations, be sure to do a patch test to ensure it is safe to use. Discard immediately any batches that may be contaminated by other ingredients, or preparations that develop mold as they could cause infections or become poisonous.

Essential oils are not recommended for use by infants and pregnant women. Children and sensitive individuals should use essential oils sparingly except for lavender and rose.

## How to Make Your Own Herbal Remedies

### Basic Equipment
- clean glass jars with metal lids, metal containers, or glass bottles that seal well (Boil them in water to sterile them if you've used them before)
- wooden spatula or spoon
- wooden chopsticks or stirrers
- sauce pot
- double boiler
- mesh strainer
- muslin cloth, cheesecloth, or coffee/oil filters
- parchment paper (optional) or paper sandwich bags
- Blender
- wooden, stone, or ceramic blending bowl
- tinted glass bottles
- droppers

### Basic Ingredients
- beeswax

- carrier oils such as olive oil, sweet almond oil, coconut oil, jojoba oil, or grapeseed oil (you can blend different ones to make one that suits your needs)
- essential oils of your choice
- dried herbs as per your choice
- raw honey
- water (distilled)
- infused oils (you can make your own or buy them)
- witch hazel water
- aloe vera
- vodka or grain alcohol 40-50% alcohol (80-90 proof)
- vodka or grain alcohol 70-100% alcohol
- fresh herbs
- glycerin (glycerol)
- apple cider vinegar

## Note: Before you make your own herbal preparations

Always do research and take notes for your preparation labels about each herb or ingredient regarding who can take it safely, and any other precautions or warnings. This is because each herb has different properties and so interacts with a person's body chemistry and medication in a different way. It is especially important to note if the herb or spice interacts with common medications and chronic health conditions such as diabetes, high blood pressure, people on blood thinners, etc.

Also, take into consideration that experimenting with different mixtures of herbs causes chemical reactions, which may give you very different properties or even produce poisonous results. Unless you are trained in herbology, it's best to stick to well-known and trusted combinations and quantities.

## Basic Salve Recipe

This salve should keep for up to one year.

1. ½ cup of two base oils or 1 cup of oil. (8 0z). Warm your base oils (coconut, olive, jojoba, grapeseed, etc.) in a saucepan or double boiler on medium heat.

2. ¼ cup each dried herb. (6 oz). Add your infused oil or dried herbs. Boil for about 20 minutes.

3. Strain any dried herbs from the oil using the cheesecloth, or another filter. Wipe off any herb detritus and add the clear oil back into the pot. If you're only using infused oil, go directly onto the next step.

4. Put the pot of oil back onto medium heat.

5. 2 Tablespoons of honey. Stir in the honey until it is completely combined.

6. ¼ cup beeswax (2 oz), in pellets or cut into pieces. Add to the heated oil. Stir continuously, so all the wax is combined.

7. Pour into the sterile glass jars or another container.

8. If you are adding essential oils, add a few drops to each jar and stir it in well with a chopstick.

9. Allow the salve to cool, occasionally stirring in the jar, so it cools evenly.

10. Seal tightly once it is thoroughly cooled.

If you would prefer a thicker consistency for the final salve, add a little more beeswax to the mixture while it is on medium heat.

## Basic Cream Recipe

This cream should keep for up to a month or a little longer if refrigerated.

1.  In a double-boiler set to medium heat, combine ¾ cup (12 oz) carrier oil (olive, coconut, jojoba, or infused oil) and ½-1 oz (2 tablespoons) beeswax. Stir continuously until the beeswax is melted.

2.  Pour the oil blend into a blender and let cool. At room temperature, it turns cloudy and is ready for the next step.

3.  Turn the blender onto high.

4.  Slowly stream 1 cup (8 oz) of distilled water or rosewater into the center of the blender's mix to emulsify the ingredients. Don't let your blender overheat as it will remelt the wax and stop the emulsification process. Allow your blender to cool down before continuing if it overheats.

5.  Stop adding water when the mix turns white and stiff.

6.  Add in essential oil—just 2 to 5 drops depending on the strength; 2 drops for strong oils and 5 drops for milder oils such as lavender and rose. Don't add too much essential oil if you're using an infused oil.

7.  Pour the cream into clean, sterile jars or containers.

**8.** Seal thoroughly.

## Basic Methods for Infusing Oil

There are four ways to infuse oil. Two require heat, and two don't. You'll know your oil is infused when it takes on the color and scent of the herb or spice. Most infused oils should be fine to use for two months up to a year. When the oil goes rancid (the smell and consistency will change) or it develops mold, it's time to discard it.

Cold Method One—4 to 6 Weeks

1. Fill a jar (mason jars are best) or bottle with a herb of your choice till it is about ⅔ full.

2. Fill the bottle to the top with olive oil or another carrier such as coconut oil. Ensure all the herbs are covered.

3. Store in a cool, dark place for the next 4 to 6 weeks.

4. Shake the bottle often.

5. When the oil is done, strain the herbs out using cheesecloth or a coffee filter.

6. Decant into sterile glass bottles, label and store in a cool place or refrigerate.

Cold Method Two—Just over 24 hours

1. Smash or grind 1 oz (28g) of dried herbs into a rough powder. Place in a jar or bottle.

2. Pour a ½ oz (15 ml) of whole grain alcohol such as vodka into the bottle.

3. Shake the jar or mix the herbs and alcohol until the herbs look like damp soil.

4. Leave to steep for 24 hours.

5. Place herbs in a blender. Add at least 8 oz (1 cup) of carrier oil of your choice. Add more oil to cover the herbs if necessary.

6. Blend for about 5 minutes.

7. Strain the oil into a glass container, then decant for storage. Label the oil and expected expiration date.

Warm Method One—2 to 4 weeks

This method uses the same process as Cold Method One, but instead of leaving it in the pantry or other cool, dark place, we place it in the sun. Stand the infusing jar or bottle on a sunny windowsill or another sunny spot. Shake the bottle every now and then. The oil should be infused in two to four weeks. The longer you leave it on the windowsill, the stronger your infusion will be.

NB! Take care with the carrier oil you use for this method. Olive oil and coconut oil work best, while other oils such as grapeseed or rosehip oil may spoil. Covering the bottle with a paper bag or using smoked bottles may get you the best results.

Warm Method Two—Between 30 minutes and three days

This method requires a stove or crockpot.

1. Place 8 oz (1 cup) carrier oil and 6 oz (¼ cup) dried herbs in a saucepan, a double boiler, or a crockpot. Ensure the herbs are fully covered and that they are about 2 inches (5 cm) over the herbs.

2. Either place the herbs over a low heat 100 F (37 C) for 1 to 5 hours or on medium heat for about

20 minutes, ensuring the herbs aren't frying. If you have the time, you can leave the infusing oil on a constant heat of low in a crockpot for 48 to 72 hours to get a more potent infusion.

3. Allow the oil to cool, then strain using a filter or cheesecloth.

4. Decant into sterile glass bottles or jars and label with contents, date produced and expected expiration date.

## Tinctures and Tonics

Tinctures and tonics are much the same as infusions, except that a tincture is always made with an alcohol or glycerin base.

They are usually administered by a dropper as it's important to only ingest small amounts of tinctures. The usual safe daily dosage is usually 2,5ml or ½ a teaspoon twice a day. Tinctures can be diluted in water, in tea, in fruit juice, or even in sparkling water.

Store tinctures in small tinted bottles to keep them longer.

Basic Tincture Method Using Alcohol

Alcohol-based tinctures can keep up to four to five years if stored well in a cool, dry place out of sunlight.

1. Fill a mason jar with dried herbs—not too coarse—until the jar is about ½ full.

2. Add the alcohol until the jar is full and all the herbs are entirely covered.

3. Ensure there is not too much air between the lid and the alcohol.

4. Cover the top of the jar with a paper sandwich bag or parchment paper.

5. Close the jar with a metal lid, so it is airtight.

6. Gently shake the bottle so the herbs can float in the liquid.

7. Store the jar in a pantry or other cool, dark area.

8. Shake the jar a few times each day.

9. Check that the herbs are always completely covered by alcohol as they may evaporate. If the alcohol level drops, top it up with as much alcohol as required.

10. Your tincture should be ready in about 6-8 weeks.

11. Strain the herbs with cheesecloth or a mesh strainer and funnel them into a tinted bottle.

12. Label the tincture carefully and use sparingly. Include a list of herbs used and the alcohol details on each label. Also include directions for use.

Note: If you are using fresh herbs, fill the jar to about ⅔ full, then add alcohol to fill the rest of the jar. Ensure fresh herbs are finely chopped.

Tincture Method Using Glycerin or Apple Cider Vinegar

If you would like an alcohol-free tincture, glycerin provides a sweeter and more palatable alternative but will spoil faster. Glycerin-based tinctures will keep for just over a year.

Another alcohol-free option is to use the recipe above and substitute the alcohol with apple cider vinegar.

1. Mix ¾ cup vegetable glycerin with ¼ cup distilled or boiled water. Set aside.

2. Half fill a jar with dried herbs. If you're using fresh herbs, chop finely and fill the jar about ⅔ full.

3. Add the glycerin mixture into the jar, ensuring the jar is filled and the herbs are fully covered.

4. Store the bottle in a cool, dry place such as a pantry.

5. Shake the bottle every day.

6. After 4-6 weeks, your tincture is ready.

7. Strain all plant material out using a mesh strainer or coffee filter.

8. Funnel the tincture into tinted bottles.

9. Label with all the details: date bottled, ingredients, glycerin to water ratio, dosage instructions, and expected expiry date.

To make a tonic, dilute a tincture in distilled water, or add 2.5ml to a glass of juice, or tea of your choice.

## Bruises and Scrapes Salve

For use on scrapes, minor cuts, and minor burns, diaper rash, and eczema.

You will need basic ingredients of the Basic Salve recipe, with these substitutes for the herbs and essential oil.

- 6 oz (¼ cup) comfrey, dried
- 6 oz (¼ cup) calendula, dried
- 6 oz (¼ cup) oregon grape root (optional)

- 5 to 10 drops lavender essential oil

To make it: Use the basic salve recipe and use a ¼ cup of dried herbs to every ½ cup or carrier oil.

## Sunscreen

Any natural sunscreen needs to contain either zinc oxide or titanium dioxide to effectively block the sun's rays. Otherwise, you will have a sun filter cream instead of a sunblock cream. It is also hard to determine the efficiency of DIY Sunscreen as the UVB/UVA filtering will differ greatly depending on ingredients used and blends. Therefore, SPF factors will be variable. Also, homemade sunscreens are not waterproof. Therefore, further steps to prevent and minimize sunburn must be taken. The best sun protection remains covering up.

You will need:

- 1 cup shea butter
- ¼ cup jojoba oil or sweet almond oil (carrier oil)
- ¼ cup pure aloe vera (minimum 50% aloe vera)
- 2 to 3 tablespoons zinc oxide, powdered
- 25 drops of walnut extract oil

To make it:

1. In a double-boiler or saucepan, heat the shea butter, carrier oil, and walnut extract oil over medium heat.

2. Remove from heat when all the shea butter is melted and all the oils are well combined.

3. Allow the oil mixture to cool.

4. When cool, stir in aloe vera.

5. When the mixture is thoroughly cooled, stir in zinc oxide until it's all well combined.

6. Decant into jars or sterile containers for use.

Note: To have a thicker sunscreen cream, add in some beeswax. To make a spray instead of a cream, leave out the shea butter, adding more carrier oil, and once the oils have cooled, add more aloe vera until you can spray from a bottle easily.

## Witch Hazel Wipes

Witch Hazel is a great antiseptic, antibacterial, antifungal, astringent, antimicrobial, and anti-inflammatory. Using wipes to help clean scrapes, cuts, bruises, and around open wounds is a swift and easy solution. These can also be used to treat sunburn, hemorrhoids, stings, and insect bites, and minor rashes.

These wipes might dry out after a few weeks, so it's best to use them quickly.

You will need:

- witch hazel (store-bought or infuse your own)
- essential oil of your choice. Lavender, peppermint, lemongrass, basil, rosemary or sage work well.
- aloe vera gel (optional)
- cotton cosmetic pads or cotton rounds
- airtight storage jar or container, or resealable airtight plastic bag

To make it: Mix the 4 to 6 drops of essential oil into about 2 oz (¼ cup) with hazel. Add 1 oz (30ml) of aloe vera to the solution if you are using it. Place the cotton swabs and wipes in the airtight container. Gently pour the solution over the wipes. Ensure the swabs are wet through, but not to the point of dripping. Seal the container.

Note: You can also infuse witch hazel much as you infuse oil by using Cold Method One. However, the infusion is best refrigerated and may not be suitable for long-term storage in a first aid kit. It would be best used to treat rashes and other short-term irritations topically for a few days.

## Anti-Itch Salve

You will need basic ingredients of the Basic Salve recipe, with these substitutes for the herbs and essential oil.

- plantain infused oil (make your own or store-bought)
- essential oils. Lavender, lemongrass, tea tree oil, and peppermint work well

To make it: Follow the Basic Salve Recipe, skipping the addition of herbs and the straining of the oil. Once the infused oil is heated, skip straight to adding in the beeswax.

Note: The addition of peppermint, lemongrass, basil, or lavender, may also work as an insect repellent for certain insects such as centipedes and wasps.

## Burn Salve

You will need: basic ingredients of the Basic Salve recipe with these substitutes and additions. It's best to use coconut oil for this recipe.

- Additional raw honey
- aloe vera

- lavender essential oil (optional)

To make it: Heat ½ cup (4 oz) coconut oil on medium heat. Stir in ¾ cup (6 oz) of honey. Add 1 to 2 oz of beeswax to get to the consistency you desire. Stir until the beeswax has melted. Pour oil into a dish to cool. When the oil is cool, stir in 2 to 4 oz of aloe vera. Add essential oil. Stir slowly and thoroughly. Decant into storage jars or containers and label.

## Rash Cream

You will need: basic ingredients of the Basic Cream recipe, with these substitutes for the herbs and essential oil.

- ⅓ cup aloe vera
- ¾ cup infused oil of marshmallow root, chamomile, and lemon balm. Optional herbs or substitute herbs could be calendula or lavender
- 1 to 2 drops of essential oil. Tea tree oil, lavender, or peppermint work well
- ⅔ cup distilled water

To make it: Heat the infused oil and the beeswax and stir until the beeswax has melted. Remove from heat. When the oil is at room temperature, combine the water and aloe vera. Slowly blend the water into the oil using a blender as in the Basic Cream recipe. Once the emulsification is done, add in the essential oil. Decant into jars or containers and label the cream.

## Peppermint Tincture

Peppermint is great for treating abdominal pains, indigestion and helping relieve headaches. It is also antibacterial. However, care must be taken if a person is on medication as it does interact with a range of medications. While peppermint can also be applied topically to help relieve congestion (as you do with a salve), children and infants should not be administered peppermint at all.

To make peppermint tincture, follow the basic tincture recipe of your choice.

## Disinfectant and Hand Sanitizers

If you run out of disinfectants or hand sanitizers, you can also make your own. However, they may not be as effective as approved store-bought products, but they are useful in a bind. These recipes are particularly helpful if you are in a remote location or your area is under an extended general quarantine.

Some of the ingredients in these recipes may damage or stain unsealed surfaces such as granite or wood. However, they are good for disinfecting daily items if no bleach is available.

NB! These recipes contain alcohol and are highly flammable! Store safely away from heat sources. Store them in child-safe places.

## Disinfectant Spray

You will need:

- ½ cup white distilled vinegar
- 1 ½ cup alcohol (highest proof Vodka available or rubbing alcohol that is a minimum of 70% proof)
- 50 drops lavender or tea tree essential oil

To make it: Combine the essential oil and alcohol in a large enough spray bottle. Shake the bottle to mix the two thoroughly. It is best to use a figure-eight motion. Then add the vinegar and mix thoroughly again. The disinfectant is now ready for use.

## Two Step Bleach-free Disinfecting

You will need:

- hydrogen peroxide
- white distilled vinegar
- a spray bottle
- a spray cap to fit the hydrogen peroxide bottle if possible

Warning! Never mix hydrogen peroxide and vinegar together in a bottle! The fumes released when they are combined are poisonous and can damage your health.

How to do it: First use the hydrogen peroxide on a surface by spraying it. Let it lie for about 5 minutes. Wipe off the area thoroughly. Next, spray on the vinegar. Let it lie for about another 5 minutes. Then wipe off the vinegar. The surface is now disinfected of the most common illness-causing organisms.

## Hand Sanitizer Method One

Remember to wash your hands first, as the disinfectant cannot do its job through dirt, grease and other oils. If no water is available, wipe your hands down first with antibacterial wipes such as the witch hazel wipes.

Ensure the alcohol you're using isn't diluted so that the 60-70% alcohol concentration is maintained in the end product.

When mixing hand sanitizers, ensure the surface you're working on is disinfected, as well as your hands and all the equipment you're using.

Don't touch the hand sanitizer liquid when decanting it into bottles. Allow the bottles to sit for 72 hours if possible.

You will need:

- ½ cup aloe vera gel

- 1 cup ethanol or isopropyl alcohol (rubbing alcohol 99% proof)

- 10-20 drops of essential oil. Peppermint, cloves, lavender, or tea tree oil work well. Lemon juice can be substituted for essential oils

To make it: Mix the essential oil into the aloe vera gel in a large plastic bottle or a bucket. Add the alcohol. Mix thoroughly or, if it's in a bottle, shake the bottle gently. Decant the sanitizer into a bottle with a screw cap or a hand dispenser. If you'd like to use this recipe for a spray, add a little more undiluted alcohol until you get a spraying consistency.

Note: To make this sanitizer in larger or smaller quantities, simply stick to the 1 part aloe vera to 2 parts 99% proof alcohol.

## Hand Sanitizer Method Two

You will need:

- ½ cup alcohol highest proof vodka (100% or over) or rubbing alcohol (99%)

- 1 tsp vegetable glycerin (also called glycerine or glycerol)

- 10-20 drops of essential oils. Lavender, spruce, lemon, citrus, eucalyptus, or chamomile all work well

To make it: Mix the glycerin and essential oils well together in a 4 oz bottle. Add the alcohol until the bottle is full. Cap the bottle and shake gently to mix.

## Alternatives to the First Aid Kit Material

## Burns

- If you don't have water to cool the burn, use any other cool liquid such as juice, beer, milk, etc. Any harmless liquid will do as your priority is to cool the area until you have access to cold, running water.

- Remember, the burn should be cooled for at least twenty minutes for the treatment to be effective.

- If you don't have cling film to cover the burn, use a clean plastic bag such as a carrier bag, freezer bag, sandwich bag, or similar. These items won't stick to the burn and will prevent infection.

- Plastic bags are well suited to covering a burned hand or foot.

## Broken Bones

If you don't know what padding to use for broken bones, use clothing, blankets, etc. Or hold the injured part yourself. A half-rolled magazine held by duct tape can serve as a makeshift cast or protection for a limb for short-term transport. Popsicle sticks make good finger splints.

## Heavy Bleeding

If you don't have dressing pads to put on the wound, use a clean t-shirt, or clean tea towel, sanitary pads, or clamp the person's hand over their injury.

Your priority is to put pressure on the wound to stop or slow down the bleeding.

## Diabetic Emergency

If you don't have glucose tablets, use orange juice, a few sugar cubes, candy, or packets of sugar. Alternatively, use any regular fizzy drink, except diet beverages.

## Head Injury

If you don't have any ice cubes, use a packet of frozen peas wrapped in a tea towel. Alternatively, use clothing soaked in cold water and wrung out. A half-collapsed baseball cap can be used as a temporary neck brace. Push the back of the cap in so the front of the cap with the peak creates a cradle (just as many stores stack them). Fit the cap with the peak facing the person's chest so that the rest of the cap cradles their chin. Secure the cap with duct tape.

## Eye Injury

Use a paper cup to protect the eye if no eye shield is available. Secure it with duct tape. Ensure you don't tape over hair, if possible.

# Hypothermia

If there are no blankets or space blankets available, consider using aluminum foil if it is at hand.

# Conclusion

Well done! You're now equipped to face and help a distressed person through a variety of emergencies.

You have your list of items and medication you can either buy and sometimes make yourself for your first aid kits and responses. In fact, you have more than one method to handle skin infections and promote healing. You can even improvise aids like a sling or a splint when needed.

You have your steps to follow in both minor and major emergencies, whether an insect bite, a minor burn, or a major burn or hypothermia. You even know how to identify and treat emergencies related to chronic illnesses, such as a person experiencing a heart attack or suffering from hypoglycemia.

Most importantly, you know to keep calm, how to keep yourself safe while assisting someone, and how to manage the situation until professional help arrives.

Your next step is to get certified in first aid techniques such as CPR or expanding your knowledge in preparing natural remedies that are safe and effective for home and first-aid use.

We like to keep a batch of multi-purpose herbal salves such as the Bruises and Cuts Salve on hand for everyday use. We also encourage you to experiment with these homemade preparations, so you have one that is uniquely suited to your and your family's needs.

As a parting note, we'd like you to keep some things in mind.

# Remember

Communicate with the person you're treating from the moment you approach them. This will reassure both of you. Explain what you intend to do—the treatment—and tell them what you're doing at each step unless you're doing CPR. Keep your voice low and steady, and if they are agitated, this will also help them calm down and follow any instructions you may need to give them.

Use gentleness to attend to younger children and babies. Treat them as fragile and try not to let your sense of urgency result in your use of forceful movements when dealing with them. Children may need more reassurance and patience if they are conscious. It will be worth taking a moment to talk to them and explain that you mean no harm, and only want to help them. If their parent or an older sibling is present, let them talk to the child. Keep your voice calm and friendly while working with the child and don't let them sense any worry you might feel about their condition.

Only use medication from a first aid kit that has not expired and herbal remedies that still smell good.

# Self-care

Self-care is vitally important before, during, and after you've given first aid in an emergency. After all, if you are ill or experiencing extreme anxiety throughout, you cannot be as effective as you'd like to be or help as you might wish.

Before you begin attending to a person in distress, do all you can to ensure your safety as well as theirs. For instance, if you have a bright jacket or flashlight, it's a good idea to use it or turn it on if you are attending to someone in dim light at the side of the road. Or if you're helping someone in freezing weather, you can also take a minute to wear your down coats and pull on a hat or beanie and wear gloves, so you don't get frostbite or worse. Also, be aware of your physical limitations and your own needs. Don't be afraid to ask for help from bystanders or others present. For example, if you are petite and a giant of a person is choking, don't attempt the Heimlich maneuver. Thump their back between the shoulder blades instead or call the attention of someone bigger in stature to assist.

While you're attending the person, no one expects you to be super-human. Do the best you can, but if you're exhausted and can't continue chest compressions, it's okay to take a break and let someone else take over, or if you're alone, to try reviving the person again if you feel that's possible. When you've done your best, there's nothing else anyone can ask of you.

If you fear contamination or have a cold, it's okay to ask a conscious person in distress to help dress their wound. Always wear gloves and other protective gear if you have them available. Use a pocket mask or face mask where possible if you're giving CPR.

If you feel you can't do a technique, look for help or a safe alternative. Remember, your priority is to preserve life, prevent deterioration, and promote recovery. Your priority isn't about getting top marks in a book exam.

During and after your care of the person, practicing breathing or relaxation techniques will help you stay calm and keep you alert and focused.

After the incident, you may run through a range of emotional responses to your experience and even that of the person, particularly if you are very empathetic. This is normal. If the feelings of wellbeing, confidence, and gratitude continue, know that you've earned them and enjoy them. However, if you feel anxiety, are hyper alert, experience nightmares, stress, other negative emotions, or take on the experience of the person that you've helped, you need to talk to someone to fully process the experience and find your balance again.

Discuss your experience with a good friend, your doctor or other professional. If you are in contact with someone else who was at the scene, you can help each other process through your feelings and responses. If you have no one to talk to, journal your experiences and your responses.

For the next few days or weeks after the incident, ensure you get enough sleep, avoid alcohol and caffeine, and eat healthily. Exercise will help you find your balance as well.

## A Final Note

We'd like to take this opportunity to acknowledge your bravery and resilience. Stepping up to assist a distressed person takes courage as well as knowledge. Your quick actions can not only help the distressed person or save their life, but your care and observation also assist the medical professionals who will eventually arrive to take over the situation, and for this, we thank you.

We also thank you for making the world a better place for us all. While we at Small Footprint Press do our best to help everyone prepare for emergencies and prevent as many as possible from happening, we like knowing there are people out there, like you, willing to lend a helping hand when needed.

Go well and be safe!

\*\*\*

If you've found this book helpful, please leave a review on Amazon.

# References

Ames, H., & Bell, A. M. (2020, December 11). *Can you sleep with a concussion? What happens and when to seek help.* www.medicalnewstoday.com. https://www.medicalnewstoday.com/articles/can-you-sleep-with-a-concussion?c=613291398967

Angie. (2014, February 28). Chinese medicine first aid - Part one: Nosebleeds, conjunctivitis & burns. Angie Savva Acupuncture. https://www.angiesavva.com/blog/chinese-medicine-first-aid-part-one-nosebleeds-conjunctivitis-burns

*Are you prepared for a medical emergency?* (2018, January 1). Harvard Health. https://www.health.harvard.edu/staying-healthy/are-you-prepared-for-a-medical-emergency

*Basic first aid procedures - Quick tips #207 - Grainger KnowHow.* (2016, January 7). https://www.grainger.com/know-how/health/medical-and-first-aid/first-aid/kh-safety-basic-first-aid-procedures-207-qt

Beatty, K. (n.d.). Natural first aid kit. Simple Tens; Simple Tens-Karla Beatty. Retrieved June 28, 2021, from https://www.simpletens.com/natural-first-aid-kit.html

Borke, J., Zieve, D., Conaway, B., & ADAM Medical Editorial Team. (2019). *Recognizing medical emergencies: MedlinePlus Medical Encyclopedia.* Medlineplus.gov. https://medlineplus.gov/ency/article/001927.htm

Caraway: Uses, side effects, dose, health benefits, precautions & warnings. (n.d.). EMedicineHealth; WebMD Inc. Retrieved July 3, 2021, from https://www.emedicinehealth.com/caraway/vitamins-supplements.htm

Chappell, S., & Stevens, C. (2019, February 21). *A beginner's guide to making herbal salves and lotions.* Healthline. https://www.healthline.com/health/diy-herbal-salves

Cheong, T. (2019). *How to survive an asthma attack if you're caught without your inhaler.* Healthxchange.sg. https://www.healthxchange.sg/asthma/complications-management/survive-asthma-without-inhaler

Cirino, E., & Carter, A. (2019, August 28). What is a Tincture? Herbal Recipes, Uses, Benefits, and Precautions. Healthline. https://www.healthline.com/health/what-is-a-tincture#summary

Dave. (2014, July 10). *Homemade: Plantain anti-itch salve and lotion bars.* Happy Acres Blog. https://happyacres.blog/2014/07/09/homemade-plantain-anti-itch-salve-and-lotion-bars/

Emergency Responders: Tips for taking care of yourself. (2018). CDC.gov. https://emergency.cdc.gov/coping/responders.asp

Emily. (2018, March 14). *Natural, homemade postpartum wipes and cooling spray. naturally free.* https://www.naturallyfreelife.com/natural-diy-tucks-wipes-and-postpartum-cooling-spray/

Engineer, R. (2018, August 8). *Be prepared: 10 Common medical Emergencies & How to Deal With Them.* The Better India. https://www.thebetterindia.com/155315/first-aid-medical-emergencies-news/

Eske, J., & Chauvoustie, C. T. (2020, December 8). *Too much hydrogen peroxide in ear: Risks, safety, treatment, and more.* www.medicalnewstoday.com. https://www.medicalnewstoday.com/articles/too-much-hydrogen-peroxide-in-ear#risks

*First aid basics and DRSABCD. (2012).* Vic.gov.au. https://www.betterhealth.vic.gov.au/health/conditionsand treatments/first-aid-basics-and-drsabcd

*First-aid kits: Stock supplies that can save lives.* (2018). Mayo Clinic; https://www.mayoclinic.org/first-aid/first-aid-kits/basics/art-20056673

Fisher, S. (2020, October 23). *Clean naturally with these best DIY disinfectants.* The Spruce. https://www.thespruce.com/best-diy-disinfectants-4799867

Fletcher, J., & Cobb, C. (2019, June 7). *9 Home remedies for burns and scalds.* www.medicalnewstoday.com. https://www.medicalnewstoday.com/articles/319768#how-severe-is-the-burn

Fletcher, J., & Whitworth, G. (2020, January 9). *How to stop heart palpitations: 7 Home remedies and tips.* Www.medicalnewstoday.com. https://www.medicalnewstoday.com/articles/321541?c=1339616399082#home-remedies

*Frostbite: Causes, symptoms, stages, treatment & prevention.* (n.d.). Cleveland Clinic; Cleveland Clinic. Retrieved July 1, 2021, from https://my.clevelandclinic.org/health/diseases/15439-frostbite

Get Licensed UK. (2021). *Basic first aid training UK (Updated 2021).* Www.youtube.com; Get Licensed UK. https://www.youtube.com/watch?v=ErxKDbH-iiI

Gillen, D. (2013, August 23). The wonders of witch hazel - A must have for your first aid preparations. PreparednessMama. https://preparednessmama.com/wonders-of-witch-hazel/

Glenn. (2015, January 29). *Top 11 natural/alternative medicine emergency first aid items. emergency food NZ.*

https://freezedriedemergencyfood.co.nz/top-11-natural-medicine-emergency-first-aid-items/

GUIDE TO LOCAL PRODUCTION: WHO-RECOMMENDED HANDRUB FORMULATIONS. (n.d.). https://www.who.int/gpsc/5may/Guide_to_Local_Production.pdf?ua=1

Hammett, E. (2019). The latest advice on burns. BDJ Team, 6(10), 16–18. https://doi.org/10.1038/s41407-019-0186-3

Healthline Editorial Team, & Luo, E. K. (2015, September 26). *Concussion: Symptoms, diagnosis, and treatments. Healthline.* https://www.healthline.com/health/concussion?c=1600259764957#longterm-effects

Healthwise Staff, Bladh, W. H., Thompson, E. G., Husney, A., & Romito, K. (n.d.). *Chest problems | Michigan Medicine.* www.uofmhealth.org. Retrieved July 2, 2021, from https://www.uofmhealth.org/health-library/cstpn#hw86215

Healthwise Staff, Blahd, W. H., Husney, A., & Romito, K. (n.d.). *Head Injury, Age 4 and Older | Michigan Medicine.* www.uofmhealth.org. Retrieved July 1, 2021, from https://www.uofmhealth.org/health-library/hdinj#hw93594

Healthwise Staff, Blahd, W. H., Husney, A., & Romito, K. (2020a, February 26). *Dealing with emergencies | Michigan Medicine.* www.uofmhealth.org. https://www.uofmhealth.org/health-library/emerg#hw154557

Healthwise Staff, Blahd, W. H., Husney, A., & Romito, K. (2020b, February 26). *Shock | Michigan Medicine.*

www.uofmhealth.org.
https://www.uofmhealth.org/health-library/shock#tp16305

Healthwise Staff, Blahd, W. H., Romito, K., & Husney, A. (2018). *Poisoning: Home treatment.* Mayo Clinic; https://www.uofmhealth.org/health-library/poins#tw9579

Healthwise Staff, Blahd, W. H., Romito, K., Husney, A., Thompson, E. G., O' Connor, H. M., & Gabica, M. J. (2020, February 26). *Burns and electric shock | Michigan Medicine.* www.uofmhealth.org. https://www.uofmhealth.org/health-library/burns#hw109096

Healthwise Staff, Romito, K., & Husney, A. (n.d.). *How to stop bleeding.* www.uofmhealth.org. Retrieved July 1, 2021, from https://www.uofmhealth.org/health-library/zm6160#zm6160-sec

Healthwise Staff, Romito, K., Husney, A., & Gabica, M. J. (2018, August 8). *Splinting.* The Better India. https://www.uofmhealth.org/health-library/sid41216#sid41216-sec

Healthwise Staff, Thompson, E. G., Husney, A., Gabica, J., & Ryan, L. (2020, September 23). *Taking a pulse (Heart Rate) | Michigan Medicine.* Www.uofmhealth.org. https://www.uofmhealth.org/health-library/hw201445#hw201445-sec

Heidi. (2020, September 14). *DIY herb-infused witch hazel.* Blog.mountainroseherbs.com. https://blog.mountainroseherbs.com/herb-infused-witch-hazel

*Here are your survival kit essentials.* (2019). Mayo Clinic; https://www.mayoclinic.org/first-aid/emergency-essentials/basics/art-20134335

Higuera, V., & Han, S. (2017, November 13). *What to do when someone is having a stroke.* Healthline. https://www.healthline.com/health/stroke-treatment-and-timing/dos-and-donts

Hill, A., & Butler, N. (2019, December 6). *Caraway: Nutrients, benefits, and uses.* Healthline. https://www.healthline.com/nutrition/caraway#bottom-line

*How to make homemade hand sanitizer.* (n.d.). Franciscan Missionaries of Our Lady Health System. https://fmolhs.org/coronavirus/coronavirus-blogs/how-to-make-homemade-hand-sanitizer

Iftikhar, N., & Morrison, W. (2018, November 1). *Severed finger: First aid, surgery, and recovery.* Healthline. https://www.healthline.com/health/severed-finger

Iftikhar, N., & Wilson, D. R. (2019, July 23). *Benefits of fennel seeds for gas, plus how to use them.* Healthline. https://www.healthline.com/health/fennel-seeds-for-gas

Irene. (2019, August 13). How to make herb-infused oils for culinary & body care use. Blog.mountainroseherbs.com. https://blog.mountainroseherbs.com/making-herbal-oils

John Hopkins Medicine. (2019). *Acupuncture.* John Hopkins Medicine. https://www.hopkinsmedicine.org/health/wellness-and-prevention/acupuncture

Kate. (2014, June 17). *Non-Toxic DIY waterproof sunscreen.* Real Food RN. https://realfoodrn.com/diy-waterproof-sunscreen-thats-good-skin/

Krebs-Holm, L. (2019, December 20). *Ginger: Health benefits, nutrition, & how to take it.* EMediHealth. https://www.emedihealth.com/nutrition/ginger-benefits-risk

Laycock, R. (2021, February 18). Doomsday preppers: How many are preparing for the end? | Finder.com (C. Choi, Ed.). Finder.com; Finder.com/Hive Empire PTY Ltd. https://www.finder.com/doomsday-prepper-statistics

Leestma, B. (2016, April 18). *Natural disinfecting with vinegar and hydrogen peroxide.* The Make Your Own Zone. https://www.themakeyourownzone.com/homemade-disinfecting-spray-ideas/

Lindberg, S., & Weatherspoon, D. (2020, July 6). *How to Make Your Own Hand Sanitizer.* Healthline. https://www.healthline.com/health/how-to-make-hand-sanitizer#how-to-use

Lubbers, W. (2017). Emergency Procedures (C. K. Stone & R. L. Humphries, Eds.). *Access medicine; McGraw-Hill Education.* https://accessmedicine.mhmedical.com/content.aspx?bookid=2172§ionid=165057582

Mahboubi, M. (2018). *Caraway as important medicinal plants in management of diseases.* Natural Products and Bioprospecting, 9(1), 1–11. https://doi.org/10.1007/s13659-018-0190-x

*Malaria.* (n.d.). Www.who.int. Retrieved June 28, 2021, from https://www.who.int/health-topics/malaria#tab=tab_3

Marcin, A., & Wilson, D. R. (2017, March 27). *How to stop heart palpitations: 6 Home remedies and more.* Healthline. https://www.healthline.com/health/how-to-stop-heart-palpitations

Marengo, K., & Snyder, C. (2021, May 14). What Is an herbal tonic? Benefits, weight loss, and efficacy. Healthline. https://www.healthline.com/nutrition/herbal-tonic

Marr, K. (2016, December 4). *Homemade hand sanitizer spray (kid-friendly).* Live Simply. https://livesimply.me/homemade-hand-sanitizer-spray-kid-friendly/

Mayo Clinic. (2017a). *Concussion - diagnosis and treatment - mayo clinic.* Mayoclinic.org; https://www.mayoclinic.org/diseases-conditions/concussion/diagnosis-treatment/drc-20355600

Mayo Clinic. (2017b). *Concussion - Symptoms and causes.* Mayo Clinic; https://www.mayoclinic.org/diseases-conditions/concussion/symptoms-causes/syc-20355594

Mayo Clinic Staff. (n.d.-a). *First aid for food poisoning.* Mayo Clinic. Retrieved July 1, 2021, from https://www.mayoclinic.org/first-aid/first-aid-food-borne-illness/basics/art-20056689

Mayo Clinic Staff. (n.d.-b). *Foreign object in the ear: First aid.* Mayo Clinic. Retrieved July 1, 2021, from https://www.mayoclinic.org/first-aid/first-aid/basics/art-20056709

Mayo Clinic Staff. (n.d.-c). *Foreign object in the nose: First aid.* Mayo Clinic. Retrieved July 1, 2021, from https://www.mayoclinic.org/first-aid/first-aid/basics/art-20056610

Mayo Clinic Staff. (n.d.-d). *Human bites: First aid.* Mayo Clinic. Retrieved July 1, 2021, from https://www.mayoclinic.org/first-aid/first-aid-human-bites/basics/art-20056633

Mayo Clinic Staff. (2017a). *Choking: First aid.* Mayo Clinic; https://www.mayoclinic.org/first-aid/first-aid-choking/basics/art-20056637

Mayo Clinic Staff. (2017b). *Nosebleeds: First aid.* Mayo Clinic; https://www.mayoclinic.org/first-aid/first-aid-nosebleeds/basics/art-20056683

Mayo Clinic Staff. (2018a). *Electrical shock: First aid.* Mayo Clinic; https://www.mayoclinic.org/first-aid/first-aid-electrical-shock/basics/art-20056695

Mayo Clinic Staff. (2018b). *Fainting: First aid.* Mayo Clinic; https://www.mayoclinic.org/first-aid/first-aid-fainting/basics/art-20056606

Mayo Clinic Staff. (2018c). *First aid for anaphylaxis.* Mayo Clinic; https://www.mayoclinic.org/first-aid/first-aid-anaphylaxis/basics/art-20056608

Mayo Clinic Staff. (2018d). *Head trauma: First aid.* Mayo Clinic; https://www.mayoclinic.org/first-aid/first-aid-head-trauma/basics/art-20056626

Mayo Clinic Staff. (2018e). *Headache: First aid.* Mayo Clinic; https://www.mayoclinic.org/first-aid/first-aid-headache/basics/art-20056639

Mayo Clinic Staff. (2018f). *Poisoning: First aid.* Mayo Clinic; https://www.mayoclinic.org/first-aid/first-aid-poisoning/basics/art-20056657

Mayo Clinic Staff. (2018g). *Spider bites: First aid.* Mayo Clinic; https://www.mayoclinic.org/first-aid/first-aid-spider-bites/basics/art-20056618

Mayo Clinic Staff. (2018h). *Sprain: First aid.* Mayo Clinic; https://www.mayoclinic.org/first-aid/first-aid-sprain/basics/art-20056622

Mayo Clinic Staff. (2019a). *Fever: First aid.* Mayo Clinic; https://www.mayoclinic.org/first-aid/first-aid-fever/basics/art-20056685

Mayo Clinic Staff. (2019b). *Hypothermia: First aid.* Mayo Clinic; https://www.mayoclinic.org/first-aid/first-aid-hypothermia/basics/art-20056624

Mayo Clinic Staff. (2019c). *Snakebites: First aid.* Mayo Clinic; https://www.mayoclinic.org/first-aid/first-aid-snake-bites/basics/art-20056681

Mayo Clinic Staff. (2019d). *Which treatment is best for your headaches?* Mayo Clinic; https://www.mayoclinic.org/diseases-conditions/chronic-daily-headaches/in-depth/headaches/art-20047375

Mayo Clinic Staff. (2019e, July 24). *Gastroenteritis: First aid.* Mayo Clinic. https://www.mayoclinic.org/first-aid/first-aid-gastroenteritis/basics/art-20056595

Mayo Clinic Staff. (2020a, April 1). *Heatstroke: First aid.* Mayo Clinic; https://www.mayoclinic.org/first-aid/first-aid-heatstroke/basics/art-20056655

Mayo Clinic Staff. (2020b, May 30). *Sunburn: First aid.* Mayo Clinic. https://www.mayoclinic.org/first-aid/first-aid-sunburn/basics/art-20056643

McDermott, A. (2018, June 4). *First Aid for Stroke.* Healthline; Healthline Media. https://www.healthline.com/health/stroke/stroke-first-aid

McDermott, A., & Sullivan, D. (2017, April 3). *Home remedies to stop bleeding.* Healthline. https://www.healthline.com/health/home-remedies-to-stop-bleeding#witch-hazel

*Medical emergency preparation.* (n.d.). www.parentgiving.com. Retrieved June 28, 2021, from https://www.parentgiving.com/elder-care/prepare-for-a-medical-emergency/

Mental Health Commission of Canada. (n.d.). *Mental health first aid COVID-19 self-care & resilience guide.* Mental Health Commission of Canada. Retrieved July 3, 2021, from https://www.mhfa.ca/sites/default/files/mhfa_self-care-resilience-guide.pdf

Merissa. (2014, March 10). *The best burn salve recipe.* Little House Living. https://www.littlehouseliving.com/best-burn-salve.html#_a5y_p=1511158

Mrs Happy Homemaker, C. (2012, November 1). *Healing Boo-Boo Salve - aka Homemade natural neosporin.* Mrs Happy Homemaker. https://www.mrshappyhomemaker.com/healing-boo-boo-salve-a-k-a-homemade-natural-neosporin/

NHS Choices. (2019). *Asthma attacks - Asthma.* Nhs. https://www.nhs.uk/conditions/asthma/asthma-attack/

Nicholson, D. (2020, April 22). *Improvised first aid afloat.* Practical Sailor. https://www.practical-sailor.com/blog/improvised-first-aid-afloat

*Options for first aid if no first aid kit is available.* (n.d.). Redcross.org.uk; British Red Cross Society. Retrieved June 28, 2021, from https://www.redcross.org.uk/first-aid/no-first-aid-kit-no-problem

*Peppermint Oil.* (n.d.). NCCIH. https://www.nccih.nih.gov/health/peppermint-oil

Petre, A. (2018, December 19). *What Is Vegetable Glycerin? Uses, Benefits and Side Effects.* Healthline; Healthline Media. https://www.healthline.com/nutrition/vegetable-glycerin

Piazza, G. M., American College Of Emergency Physicians, & Dk Publishing, Inc. (2014). *First aid manual : the step-by-step guide for everyone.* Dk Publishing.

*Quarantine at home - coping tips | betterhealth.vic.gov.au.* (n.d.). www.betterhealth.vic.gov.au. https://www.betterhealth.vic.gov.au/health/ConditionsAndTreatments/quarantine-at-home-coping-tips

Raychel. (2017, June 13). *How to make herbal tinctures.* Blog.mountainroseherbs.com. https://blog.mountainroseherbs.com/guide-tinctures-extracts

Raypole, C., & Moawad, H. (2019, June 14). *Concussions and sleep: A dangerous mix?* Healthline. https://www.healthline.com/health/concussion-and-sleep

*Rescue Remedy drops and spray - Original Rescue Remedy.* (n.d.). Information & Sales - the Original Bach Flower Remedies; Bachflower.com. Retrieved June 28, 2021, from http://www.bachflower.com/rescue-remedy-information/

Santos-Longhurst, A., & Marcin, J. (2018, July 9). *What to Do When You or Someone You Know May Have Breathed in Too Much Smoke.* Healthline; Healthline Media. https://www.healthline.com/health/smoke-inhalation

Schauf, C. (2019, March 12). *10 Basic first aid training tips & procedures for any emergency.* Uncharted Supply Company; Uncharted Supply Company. https://unchartedsupplyco.com/blogs/news/basic-first-aid

Seladi-Schulman, J. (2019, April 25). *About peppermint oil uses and benefits.* Healthline; Healthline Media. https://www.healthline.com/health/benefits-of-peppermint-oil

SkylerRyser. (2019, February 7). *Three C's of an emergency & three P's of first aid.* Idaho Medical Academy. https://www.idahomedicalacademy.com/the-three-cs-of-an-emergency-and-the-three-ps-of-first-aid/

Stewart, J. (2015, March 23). *Hydrogen peroxide + vinegar = A disinfecting duo?* Cleaning Business Today. https://cleaningbusinesstoday.com/blog/hydrogen-peroxide-vinegar-a-disinfecting-duo/

*Stroke treatment.* (2019). Centers for Disease Control and Prevention. https://www.cdc.gov/stroke/treatments.htm

*The World's Most Natural First Aid Kit.* (2013, January 4). Redbook. https://www.redbookmag.com/body/health-fitness/advice/a14796/acupressure-points-chart/

Thompson, E. G., Gabica, M. J., Romito, K., Husney, A., & Zorowitz, R. D. (2020, March 4). *Stroke | Michigan Medicine.* www.uofmhealth.org. https://www.uofmhealth.org/health-library/hw224638#hw224684

Traditional Chinese Medicine could make "Health for One" true. (n.d.). https://www.who.int/intellectualproperty/studies/Jia.pdf

*Traveler's first aid kit.* (n.d.). www.emergencyphysicians.org. Retrieved June 28, 2021, from https://www.emergencyphysicians.org/article/health—safety-tips/travelers-first-aid-kit

Vukovich, L. (n.d.). *Make your own natural first-aid kit.* Motherearthliving.com. Retrieved June 30, 2021, from https://content.motherearthliving.com/health-and-wellness/make-your-own-natural-first-aid-kit/

Watson, K., & Wilson, D. R. (2019, July 10). Homemade sunscreens: Can you make one that is safe and effective?

Healthline.
https://www.healthline.com/health/homemade-sunscreen

WHO, I. (1997). Management of poisoning - A handbook for health care workers: Part 1 - General information on poison and poisoning: Chapter 5 - First aid: First aid for poisoning. Helid.digicollection.org. http://helid.digicollection.org/en/d/Js13469e/4.5.3.html

*You can Stop bleeding in less than 60 seconds! | Go Beyond Organic.* (2012, May 4). www.gobeyondorganic.com. http://www.gobeyondorganic.com/you-can-stop-bleeding-in-less-than-60-seconds

www.ingramcontent.com/pod-product-compliance
Lightning Source LLC
Chambersburg PA
CBHW060049100426
42742CB00014B/2745